72

Dr. Biswaroop Roy Chowdhury

DIAMOND BOOKS

BROUGHT TO YOU BY
Indo-Vietnam Medical Board

India Office:
C/o India Book of Records
B-121, 2nd Floor, Greenfields,
Faridabad -12003 (Haryana),
India
Ph. :+91-9312286540

Vietnam Office:
C/o Vietnam Book of Records
148 Hong Ha Street
9 Award, Phu Nhuan District,
Ho Chi Minh City, Vietnam
- Hotline: (+84) 903710505

Malaysia Office:
C/o Bishwaroop International Healing & Research
PT 573, Lot 15077 Jalan Tuanku Munawir,
70000 Negeri Sembilan, Malaysia
Tel :+6012-2116089

Switzerland Office:
C/o Nigel Kingsley
Kraftwerkstr. 95, ch-5465, Mellikon, Switzerland
Tel : 0041 79 222 2323

FOLLOW ME

Facebook: https://www.facebook.com/drbrc.official/

Twitter: https://twitter.com/drbrcofficial

Bitchute:https://www.bitchute.com/channel/drbiswarooproychowdhury/

Instagram: https://www.instagram.com/dr.biswarooproychowdhury/

Telegram: https://t.me/drbiswarooproychowdhury

Email: biswaroop@biswaroop.com

Website: www.biswaroop.com

Research: Rachna Sharma

Proof Reading: Sanjana Bhowmick

Coordinator: Shweta Jalhotra

Graphics Designer: Shankar Singh Koranga, Swapan Banik

Published By:

Diamond Pocket Books
X-30, Okhla Industrial Area, New Delhi-110020
Tel.:011-40712200 Email:sales@dpb.in

Delta 72 - Dr. Biswaroop Roy Chowdhury

DEDICATION

Dedicated to my angel daughter Ivy,

loving wife Neerja

&

caring parents

Shri Bikash Roy Chowdhury

Shrimati Lila Roy Chowdhury

CONTENTS

SECTION - I

SECTION - II

SECTION -I

Manufacturing Pandemic: Past, Present & Future

The Wave did not arrive as an uninvited guest, it was, orchestrated. It's not the virus. It's the meticulously scripted plan to execute what you witnessed as Wave-1 or Wave-2 and now waiting in fear for Wave-3.

Let me start by providing you with thc proof of what I just stated. Go to the end of the book and find the poster. Here you see the Covid-19 Care Hospital running under the WHO/Health Ministry guidelines, i.e., masks, PPE Kits, social distancing with the patients. The average death rate in such a centre is around 12%[1]. Now flip the poster. Here you see the 1100 bed N.I.C.E Covid-19 Centre (at Ahmednagar, Maharashtra) run by MLA Nilesh Lanke. In contrast, there is no mask, no PPE Kit, no social distancing and most importantly, zero deaths.

On one hand, in the conventional Covid-19 Centre, running under the protocol of WHO, the average cost of treatment is Rs 3.5 Lakh. The average stay in the hospital – 1 month. And most of the patients suffer from severe post-treatment side effects including, Black/White/Green (etc.) fungus, diabetes and heart disease. On the other hand, in Ahmednagar N.I.C.E Covid 19 Centre, the cost of treatment – Zero. The average stay in the N.I.C.E Centre Covid-19– 3 to 7 days,

Here no patient suffered from post-treatment side effects and based on the case study conducted on 72 patients (see the 2nd section of the book), 1/3rd of the patients were in the severe category (severity graded in accordance to ICMR guidelines)[2].

Interestingly (as you see in the second section of the book), all the severe patients were either already vaccinated for Covid-19 or were admitted as mild/moderate patients in other Covid-19 Centre/Hospital (following WHO protocol). As their condition worsened, the patient decided to shift at Ahmednagar N.I.C.E Covid-19 Centre, which follows the N.I.C.E protocol[3].

Comparing both sides of the poster, it should not be difficult for you to conclude:

Mask & Isolation Kills,

Love & Compassion Heals!

The pieces of evidence provided in this chapter will help you to conclude that the real culprit causing death is not the virus but the drugs and the treatment protocol set by our Health Ministry.

In contrast, in the N.I.C.E protocol, the most vital ingredients of the treatment were fresh air, sunlight, coconut water, citrus fruit juices and togetherness.

With the help of these ingredients, about 650 of our N.I.C.E practitioners could help recover more than 60000 Covid-19 patients with zero mortality rate and with nil post-treatment side effects. With the experience of treating more than 60000 patients completing 100 days of KISSAN N.I.C.E Camp at Delhi (Ghazipur border) with zero mortality and a case study on 72 patients, I concluded that Covid-19 is just a simple Flu/ ILI (Influenza-like-Illness), which usually infects about 20% of the population every year. However, since 2020 the entry of experimental drugs and now implementation of mass vaccination programs led to a pandemic-like situation. The adverse side effect of vaccination, as reported by at least 6%[4] of the people (translated to 2.5 crore people) and 12% excess mortality, probably as a side effect of WHO-treatment protocol, is projected as a consequence of the virus leading to now what is called the '2nd Wave'.

To prevent the upcoming imaginary '3rd Wave', or rather protect our children from this conspiracy, we have to understand our body's defence mechanism. The points mentioned below would help you understand the way our body functions and will help to remove the fear of the Delta (δ) variant or the man-made pandemic.

It all starts with a pathogen (bacteria/virus/fungi) invading our body. Our immunity, especially the primitive immunity, responds in the following manner:

Step 1: Our dendritic cells, which are present all over the body including palm (however, since last year, we tried to kill the dendritic cells by repeatedly using sanitizer), reset the thermostat of the body (located in the brain), via certain kind of proteins (cytokines/PGE2, etc.).

Step 2: Our body tries to increase its temperature. We shiver to generate heat. We shunt blood away from our arms and legs and into our core to prevent heat loss. We put on warm clothing and use hot water bottles etc.

Step 3: Now, at this high temperature, the immune cells called the Neutrophils, are performing at their peak and killing bacteria and viruses.

Step 4: Slight decrease in the oxygen level (happy hypoxia) and the triggering of inflammation in the body is part of the body's combat strategy to overcome the viral/bacterial/fungal attack.

Conclusively, an internal war is going on and the body's weapons are High Temperature (fever) + Low Oxygen (low SpO2) + Inflammation (high CRP/D-Dimer).

Any attempt to lower the temperature (with paracetamol) or increase the oxygen saturation (with external oxygen supply) and reducing inflammation (by administering corticosteroids), will sabotage the war in favor of the virus/bacteria/fungi leading to a mild/moderate patient getting converted into a severe patient, with an extended stay at the hospital, and often returning home with treatment side effects like diabetes/heart diseases/Mucormycosis (black/white fungus) and also with a high risk of mortality.

Let us imagine a scenario wherein your house is under attack and you deploy soldiers to counter attack. As the war begins, so does the unpleasant noises of the ammunition. You at this point, unable to bear the unpleasant noises, instruct your troop of soldiers to put their weapons down. As a result, there is no more deafening noise, but it doesn't mean that you have averted the danger. Your enemy is still looming around.

Similarly, it is the same scenario in your body. When your body temperature rises, it means your body is fighting a war against external enemies like viruses/bacteria/fungus. The biggest weapon your immune system has to fight these pathogens is Fever. When you consume paracetamol to reduce your temperature, you give ample opportunity to the pathogens to quickly spread and attack your body.

To date, the trial conducted on animals who were given paracetamol to lower body temperature has revealed that the animals have either died or suffered from prolonged illness.[5] The trials conducted over the past 50 years on humans who consumed paracetamol are listed below.

List of Studies/Trials on Paracetamol/Antipyretics

Year	**Place**	**Outcome (Placebo vs Paracetamol/ Antipyretics)**
1975	University of Illinois[6]	Among the experimentally infected cold virus subjects, those treated with antipyretics, shed virus from their nose significantly longer.
1989	Johns Hopkins Hospital[7]	Among the chickenpox patients, those given paracetamol, took significantly longer to heal
1990	University of Adelaide, South Australia[8]	Among the experimentally infected rhinovirus volunteer, those given antipyretic had worse congestion, running nose, sneezing, sore throat and cough.
1994	Fujimoto Children's Hospital, Japan[9]	Among the children with viral infection, those who received paracetamol were more likely to develop severe pneumonia requiring hospitalization

Year	Place	Outcome (Placebo vs Paracetamol/ Antipyretics)
2000	University of Maryland School of Medicine[10]	Among the experimentally infected influenza virus volunteers, those who were treated with antipyretics had more severe illness and lasted 3 to 4 days longer
2005	University of Miami School of Medicine[11]	Among the trauma patients, those who were given antipyretics to reduce fever were more likely to develop infection and more likely to die.
2019	Phramongkutklao College of Medicine[12]	Among the dengue patients, those given paracetamol developed severe injury including hemorrhaged and acute kidney injury

The trial reveals, whenever fever occurs due to an infection or any other ailment, consuming paracetamol or antibiotics has prolonged the illness with severe side effects or caused death.

A trial[13] conducted in 2016 on humans reveals that a person who has fever while being infected has a lesser chance of dying. Interfering with temperature by consuming medicines could prove fatal. Henceforth, do not worry about high body temperature; consider it as; your friend and not a foe.

Some people have the fear that a high fever could cause seizures and fits. Yes, in rare cases it can cause fits and seizures, which might look very scary, but be rest assured, it causes no permanent damage. On the contrary, you may think of reducing the temperature by consuming antipyretics thinking it would help to control the fits, however the study proves otherwise[14].

Contrary, there are high chances that your stay in the hospital might get prolonged and could also result in death.

Despite numerous trials and studies over the past year revealing the detrimental effects of paracetamol, our Health Ministry, in June 2021, released a treatment guideline protocol for the kids to combat the imaginary '3rd Wave' with the high dose of paracetamol. The guidelines clearly state, that if the temperature of a child crosses 100°F, then the child should be given paracetamol every 4-6 hours of interval. If you follow this deadly guideline, then a mild infection would convert to moderate, which would further become severe. The chances of the child dying not because of the infection but due to unnecessary medical interference increase manifold. (Check the guidelines given on page 18-19)

Similar to fever, sometimes the low oxygen in the body is a strategy to fight the virus, as many respiratory viruses become inactive at low oxygen levels.[15,16,17] The phenomenon of Happy Hypoxia, meaning although the oxygen saturation of the patient is on the lower side (say around 80 to 92 %), the patient does not feel breathlessness. In this case, trying to increase the SpO2 level with oxygen may amplify the severity of the patient, like causing pneumonia and other complications. If the patient shows signs of breathlessness, which is rare (could only happen if the patient was administered with antiviral), then prone ventilation and Fan Therapy should be the line of action[18].

Similarly, inflammation can be seen as the 3rd pillar of the body's defence system while fighting pathogens. Initiation of corticosteroid and anticoagulant based on the diagnostic like CRP, D-Dimer, or HRCT score can lead to more suffering and disastrous end for the patient.

The new guidelines for the treatment of Covid-19 in children as released by our Health Ministry, a cocktail of paracetamol, anticoagulant, antimicrobials, steroids and oxygen therapy, is a master plan to convert the simple flu into a severe disease to justify another lockdown in the name of the 3rd Wave. The keenness to implement the lockdown can be understood, if you read the 'Oxfam Virus Inequality Report'[19] *(released on 25th January 2021, in World Economic Forum). Lockdown*

Guidelines for Management
Ministry of Health & Family

Asymptomatic

- Suspected contact
[RAT or RTPCR negative or not available]
- Incidentally detected [RAT or RTPCR positive]

Home isolation (tele consultation SOS)

Mainstay of Treatment

- Infants and younger children to stay under immediate care of parents/guardians
- No specific medication required for COVID-19 infection
- Continue medications for other conditions, if any
- Promote COVID appropriate behaviour (mask, strict hand hygiene, physical distancing); please see guide for using mask
- Fluids and feeds: ensure oral fluids to maintain hydration and give a nutritious diet
- Advise older children and family to stay connected and engage in positive talks through phone, video- calls, etc.
- Parent/caregivers to contact the doctor in case of appearance of symptoms

Mild

- Sore throat, rhinorrhoea
- Cough without breathing difficulty
- SpO2 ≥94% on room air
- For other symptoms, see COVID-19 symptoms – at a glance

Home isolation (tele consultation SOS) or COVID Care Centre

Mainstay of Treatment

- For fever, give paracetamol 10-15mg/kg/dose; may repeat every 4-6 hours
- For cough, give throat soothing agents and warm saline gargles in older children and adolescents
- Fluids and feeds: ensure oral fluids to maintain hydration and give a nutritious diet
- No other COVID-19 specific medication needed
- Antimicrobials are not indicated
- Maintain monitoring chart including counting of respiratory rate 2-3 times a day, look for chest indrawing, cold extremities, urine output, oxygen saturation, fluid intake, activity level, especially for young children
- Promote COVID appropriate behaviour (mask, strict hand hygiene, physical distancing); please see guide for using mask
- Advise older children and family to stay connected and engage in positive talks through phone, video- calls, etc.
- Parent/caregivers to contact the doctor in case of deterioration of symptoms

# of COVID-19 in Children
Welfare Govt. of India[20]

Moderate	Severe
• In addition to symptoms in mild cases, check for pneumonia which may not be apparent • Rapid respiration (age-based): <2 months RR ≥60/min; 2-12 months, RR ≥50/min; 1-5 years, RR ≥40/min; >5 years, RR ≥30/min; AND/OR SpO2 90–93% on room air • For other symptoms, see COVID-19 symptoms – at a glance	• SpO2 <90% on room air • Any of the following – signs of severe pneumonia, acute respiratory distress syndrome, septic shock, multi-organ dysfunction syndrome, or pneumonia with cyanosis, grunting, severe retraction of chest, lethargy, somnolence, seizure • For other symptoms, see COVID-19 symptoms – at a glance
Admit in DCHC or COVID-19 Hospital	Admit in HDU/ICU of COVID-19 Hospital
Mainstay of Treatment • Initiate oxygen if SpO2 is <94% and maintain between 94–96% • Maintain fluid and electrolyte balance o Encourage oral fluids (breast feeds in infants) o Initiate intravenous fluid therapy if oral intake is poor • Corticosteroids are not required in all children with moderate illness; they may be administered in rapidly progressive disease • Fever with temperature >38°C (or 100.4°F): Paracetamol 10-15mg/kg/dose; may repeat every 4- 6 hours • Anti-microbials to be administered if there is evidence/strong suspicion of superadded bacterial infection; please see antimicrobial use guide • Supportive care for comorbid conditions, if any	**Mainstay of Treatment** • Initiate immediate oxygen therapy and maintain target SpO2 94–96% • Maintain fluid and electrolyte balance • Corticosteroids therapy to be initiated • Anticoagulants may also be indicated • Exercise caution; see use of corticosteroids and anticoagulants guide • In case Acute Respiratory Distress Syndrome (ARDS) or shock develops, initiate necessary management; see ARDS and Shock guide • Antimicrobials to be administered if there is evidence/strong suspicion of superadded bacterial infection; see antimicrobial use guide • May need organ support in case of organ dysfunction e.g. renal replacement therapy

resulted in a major economic shift benefiting a select group of people while the rest became poorer.

Here are the probable 3-steps, which could be used to manufacture the 3rd Wave.

Step 1: Diarrhoea or Pneumonia kills one child every 2 minutes in India[21]. And if we add death due to hunger/ malnutrition, it will sadly be one child every 5 seconds[22]. Although the media rarely reported on this issue in the last several years; but suddenly now the camera will zoom towards the sad reality, and your television screen will be full of these unfortunate visuals, giving an impression as if it is happening for the first time, leading to the conclusion of the arrival of the 3rd Wave.

Step 2: Millions of adverse reactions and thousands of death has already been reported as a result of the massive vaccination drive[23] for Covid-19. High chances are, a similar pursuit will be attempted on our children and all the adverse reactions may be portrayed as the consequences of the imaginary 3rd Wave.

Step 3: The panic resulting from the above two steps may prompt the parents to identify the otherwise simple seasonal cold, cough or flu as a deadly disease, and they would subject their children to the new treatment guidelines of Covid-19, resulting in mayhem. Remember, monsoon season is around the corner (July to September) and during this season, almost 100% of the children suffer from flu or cold-like symptoms, which most of the time get resolved on their own or at the most need rest and hydration to cure.

In the backdrop of continuous lockdown, resulting in joblessness, forced migration of labourers, panic by the media and heroic misinterpretation of the importance of ventilators, oxygen cylinders, vaccination, masks and the introduction of the term 'The Delta (δ) variant' is strategically camouflaging, the truth leading the masses in believing the imaginary, 3rd Wave as a potential threat.

To know the truth and to remove the media-created illusion of the pandemic, you need to be aware of few facts about viruses:

1. The primary nature of all kinds of viruses is to constantly mutate and produce a new variant, similar to all living beings' need for reproduction.

2. As in humans, like all other living beings, there may be minor characteristics that may distinguish the offspring from its parents, but those variations will never be critical enough to assume someday, humans may give birth to a creature as large as an elephant or as small as a rat. Despite all variations, humans are only capable of producing humans within a certain conceivable limit. Similarly, a variant of a particular virus is almost a copy of it.

3. To date, science has not yet progressed any closer to affirming the fact, when a particular variant or a mutant of the virus is born.

Now, with all the above facts in mind, look at the much-hyped 'The Delta (δ) variant' of SARS-CoV-2.

Let us assume that science has successfully isolated and distinguished the delta variant, as reported on 5th October 2020, for the 1st time[24]. But it should not be interpreted in any way that the Delta variant was born on 5th October 2020.

Further on 31st May 2021, it was renamed by WHO as the Delta variant (previously, it was called B-1617.2)[25]. Much media coverage followed. But remember, the magnitude of media coverage is not the parameter to estimate the severity of the variant or to ascertain a fact.

For example, Jai Hemant was a man who was renamed 'Tiger Shroff' in the year 2014 and much media publicity followed. However, it is a matter of common sense to understand that neither he was born in 2014 nor became a tiger. Yes, it is definitely, a good PR strategy, which creates an image of him having a tiger-like strength and agility to some of the unsuspecting masses.

Armed with a good PR strategy and media buying capabilities, anyone can be projected, as anything one desires to be. Amongst thousands of variants including

Alpha, Beta, Gamma, Lota, etc., this time the camera is paid to focus on the Delta variant. And the propaganda strategy is all scripted by organisations like WHO and GISAID. The Chief Scientist of WHO, Dr. Soumya Swaminathan (who propagated misinformation about HIV) and our Health Minister, Dr. Harsh Vardhan, the Chairman of the Executive Board of WHO (who ensured every child in India takes the polio drops, which is banned in the developed country, as it causes paralysis), are the people who collaborated in spreading misinformation about the current situation or specifically about the Delta variant[26].

Few of the misinformation about the Delta variant:

1. It is more infectious. And if one member gets infected, the whole family gets infected.
2. It's more deadly for children and even hypothesised that it may cause altogether a new disease amongst children, interestingly called MIS-C (Multi-System Inflammatory Syndrome in Children)[20].
3. It was first discovered in India, specifically in Maharashtra hence also termed as Indian variant.

It's all about the name game. As you have seen the climax of the man-made 2nd wave, ended with the launch of yet another new term called Black Fungus, which of course expanded to White and Green fungus and will probably use the rest of the colours from the Pantone cards, so be cautious and protect your child from getting victimised with MIS-C.

All you need to do is simply follow these 3 easy steps to escape the new season of the pandemic:

Step–I: Stop watching television, particularly news channels. Avoid reading newspapers.

Step – II: Do not decide to vaccinate your child. Vaccination has not proven to provide any protection, whatsoever against anything.[23,27,28]

Step– III: If your child suffers from cold, cough, fever (which every child is likely to suffer for about 6 times every year), let him/her be on the 3-Step Flu Diet[29] and little rest or contact us at our 24x7 helpline number given in the back cover of this book or get admitted at our free N.I.C.E. hospital/Covid-19 Centres in Indore and Ahmednagar (Maharashtra).

And also read section II, which narrates the stories of the 72 Covid-19 patients, who were part of the Case Study done in Ahmednagar N.I.C.E Covid-19 Centre. Each of the stories will bring you closer to the truth and shatter the misinformation spread by the so-called mainstream media.

I hope the truth will prevail and give you utmost freedom from fear and panic of the much-publicised 'The Delta (δ) variant'.

References

Ref 1: Repurposed antiviral drugs for COVID-19 –interim WHO SOLIDARITY trial results | New England Journal of Medicine doi: 10.1056/NEJMoa2023184

Ref 2 : AIIMS/ ICMR-COVID-19 National Task Force/Joint Monitoring Group (Dte.GHS) Ministry of Health & Family Welfare, Government of India _ CLINICAL GUIDANCE FOR MANAGEMENT OF ADULT COVID-19 PATIENTS 17th May 2021
https://www.icmr.gov.in/pdf/covid/techdoc/COVID_Management_Algorithm_17052021.pdf

Ref 3 : Book - N.I.C.E way to cure Covid-19 ; authored by Dr Biswaroop Roy Chowdhury www.biswaroop.com/nicebook

Ref 4: केवल 6% ने कोविड बैक्सीन लगाने के बाद गम्भीर साइट इफेक्ट के बारे में बताया:सर्वेक्षण- India TV Hindi News

Ref 5: animals... treated or not treated with antipyretics: M. J. Kluger, "Fever Revisited," Pediatrics 90 (1992): 720-24; J. B. Covert and W. W. Reynolds, "Survival Value of Fever in Fish," Nature 267 (1977): 43–45; Kluger, "Fever in Ectotherms"; H. V. Ellingson and P. F. Clark, "The Influence of Artificial Fever on Mechanisms of Resistance," Journal of Immunology 43 (1942): 65-83; A. Lwoff, "Factors Influencing the Evolution of Viral Diseases at the Cellular Level and the Organism," Bacterial Reviews 23 (1959): 109–24; D. Rodbard, "The Role of Regional Body Temperature in the Pathogenesis of Disease," New England Journal of Medicine 305 (1981): 808–14; E. Atkins, "Treatment of Fever," New England Journal of Medicine 309 (1983): 925.

Ref 6: E. D. Stanley, G. G. Jackson, C. Panusarn, et al., "Increased Virus Shedding with Aspirin Treatment of Rhinovirus Infection," Journal of the American Medical Association 231 (1975): 1248–51.

Ref 7: T. F. Doran, C. De Angelis, R. A. Baumgardner, et al., "Acetaminophen: More Harm Than Good for Chickenpox," Journal of Pediatrics 114 (1989): 1045-48.

Ref 8: N. M. H. Graham, C. J. Burrell, R. M.Douglas, et al., "Adverse Effects of Aspirin, Acetaminophen, and Ibuprofen on Immune Function, Viral Shedding, and Clinical Status in Rhinovirus-Infected Volunteers," Journal of Infectious Diseases 162 (1990): 1277–82.

Ref 9: T. Sugimura, T. Fujimoto, H. Motoyama, et al., "Risks of Antipyretics in Young Children with Fever Due to Infectious Disease," Acta Paediatrica Japonica 36 (1994): 375–78.

Ref 10: K. I. Plaisance, S. Kudaravalli, S. S. Wasserman, et al., "Effect of Antipyretic Therapy on the Duration of Illness in Experimental Influenza, Shigella sonnei, and Rickettsia rickettsii Infections," Pharmacotherapy 20 (2000): 1417–22.

Ref 11: C. I. Schulman, N. Namias, J. Doherty et al., "The Effect of Antipyretic Therapy Upon Outcomes in Critically Ill Patients: A Randomized, Prospective Study," Surgical Infections 6 (2005): 369–75.

Ref 12: Effect of standard dose paracetamol versus placebo as antipyretic therapy on liver injury in adult dengue infection: a multicentre randomised controlled trial. Lancet Glob Health 2019; 7: e664–70

Ref 13: Z. Rumbus, R. Matics, P. Hegyi, et al., "Fever Is Associated with Reduced Hypothermia with Increased Mortality in Septic Patients: A Meta-Analysis of Clinical Trials," PLOS One (2017), doi: 10.1371/journal. pone.0170152.

Ref 14: M. Offringa and R. Newton, "Prophylactic Drug Management for Febrile Seizures in Children," Cochrane Database Systematic Reviews (2012), doi: 10.1002/14651858.CD003031.pub2; D. S. Seinfeld and J. M. Pellock, "Recent Research on Febrile Seizures: A Review,"

Journal of Neurology and Neurophysiology (2013), doi: 10.4172/2155-9562.1000165.

Ref 15: Pipiya, T., Sauthoff, H., Huang, Y. et al. Hypoxia reduces adenoviral replication in cancer cells by downregulation of viral protein expression. Gene Ther 12, 911–917 (2005). https://doi.org/10.1038

Ref 16: Budinger GRS, Mutlu GM. Balancing the risks and benefits of oxygen therapy in critically III adults. Chest. 2013;143(4):1151-1162. doi:10.1378/chest.12-1215

Ref 17: Studies With Human Influenza Virus Cultivated In Artificial Medium By T. P. Magill, M.D., Am) Thomas Francis, Jl~., M.D. (From the Hospital of The Rockefeller Institute for Medical Research)

Ref 18: Book दूसरी लहर का सच by Dr Biswaroop Roy Chowdhury www.biswaroop.com/secondwave

Ref 19 : Oxfam Inequality Virus Report- https://biswaroop.com/oxfam/

Ref 20: Comprehensive Guidelines for Management of COVID 19 in Children (below 18yrs) Ministry of Health & Family WelfareGovernment of India https://www.mohfw.gov.in/pdf/

Ref 21: Despite Better Immunisation, Diarrhoea or Pneumonia Kills 1 Child Every 2 Minutes In India: Indiasend, 15 Nov, 2018

Ref 22 : How many child deaths will it take to stop hunger? The pioneer/ Wednesday, 30 September 2020 | AR Sindhu

Ref 23: COVID-19 Vaccine side effect, www.biswaroop.com/sideeffect

Ref 24: WHO has not termed B.1.617 as Indian variant, says Centre | Hindustan Times

Ref 25: Tracking SARS-CoV-2 variants- WHO
https://www.who.int/en/activities/tracking-SARS-CoV-2-variants/

Ref 26 : Coronavirus Strain Found in India Is a 'Variant of Concern,' WHO Says. Wall Street Journal Updated May 10, 2021 4:47 pm ET

Ref 27: Covid 1981 Book authored by Dr Biswaroop Roy Chowdhury : www.biswaroop.com/covid1981

Ref 28: COVID-19 vaccine efficacy and effectiveness—the elephant (not) in the room - The Lancet Microbe Published April 20, 2021

Ref 29: www.biswaroop.com/nicecure

SECTION -II

The Case Study

Recently, Maharashtra was at the centre-stage of the world media as if it was the place where the monster is born, who can potentially wipe out the human race particularly the children. It was given a name of the "Indian Variant". This was the time when our N.I.C.E. team were working at Ahmednagar (N.I.C.E) Covid Centre, Maharashtra. I and the Covid Centre director MLA Sh. Nilesh Lanke decided to conduct a 'Scientific evidence-based case study' on one of group of Covid-19 patients and make available the well documented case study for the public, the press and the govt. authorities.

The Case study shared ahead in this book consist of 72 Covid-19 patients with 1/3rd categorized as severe patients with lowest SpO2 being 35% and highest HRCT score 20, interestingly, all the severe patients were either recently vaccinated or the one who escaped from the neighboring hospitals, when their health deteriorated while admitted there. I hope, their stories will protect you from the scare and the conspiracy of the Indian Variant aka B-16.17.2 aka Delta (δ) variant.

The case study was completed and documented in the presence of officers appointed by National Institute of Naturopathy, Pune/Ministry of Ayush/GOI:

1. Dr. Jyoti Kumbhar
2. Dr. Praveen C
3. Mr. Manoj Gupta (Volunter)
4. Mr. Sunil Singh (Volunter)

Case study at a glance

Address: Sharaddchandraji Pawar Saheb Arogya Mandir A/p-Bhalvani, Tal-Parner, Distt- Ahmednagar, Maharashtra

Centre Incharge : MLA Shri Nilesh Dnyandev Lanke

Date : 25th May, 2021 to 3rd June 2021

No of Patients : 72

Supervision by : Dr Biswaroop Roy Chowdhury (Virtually)

Medical Team (N.I.C.E Expert) :

1. Avinash Popatrao Sabare
2. Santosh Sarkale
3. Chitra Jain
4. Prateek Joshi
5. Amit Shimpi
6. Seema Mannikoth
7. Suresh v Garad
8. Vaishnavi Walnuj

		Male/Female
No of Patients	72	40/32
%		56 / 44

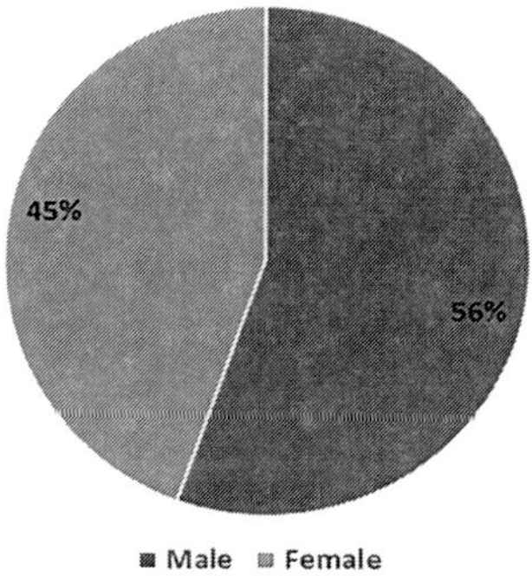

		Agc (Ycars) **≤ 17/18 to 59/≥ 60**
No of Patients	72	5/54/13
%		7/75/18

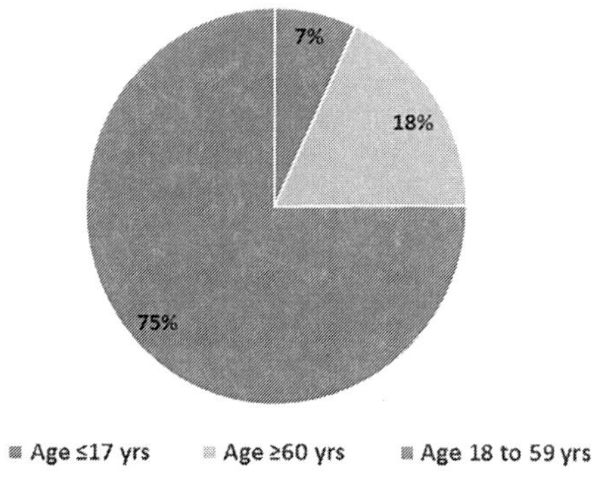

		Severe/Moderate/ Asymptomatic
No of Patients	72	14/58/0
%		20/80/0

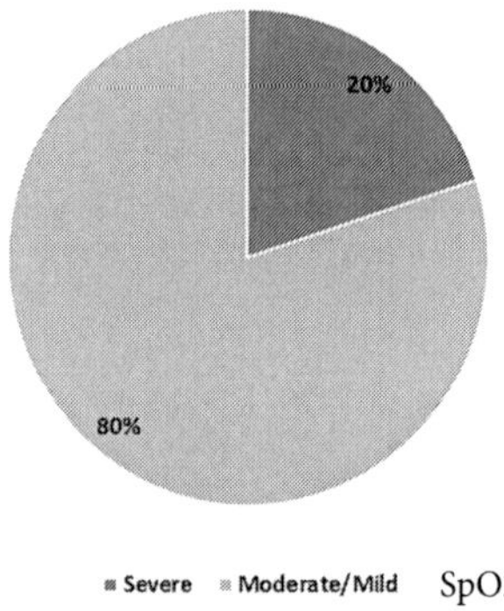

SpO2>90%

		HRCT>10
No of Patients	72	17
%		24

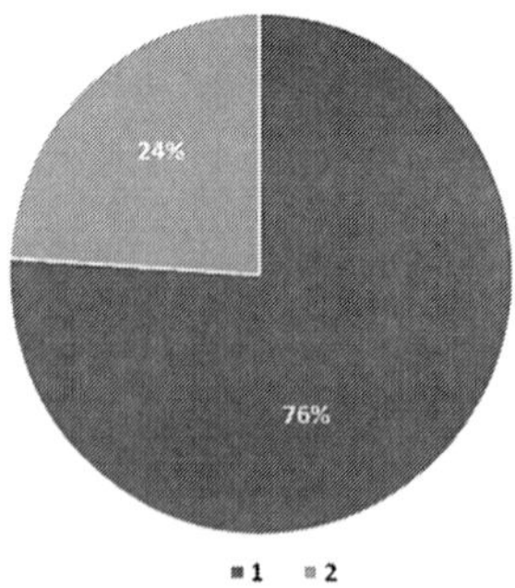

High risk patients : 25

(SPo2 < 90 or / and HRCT>10)

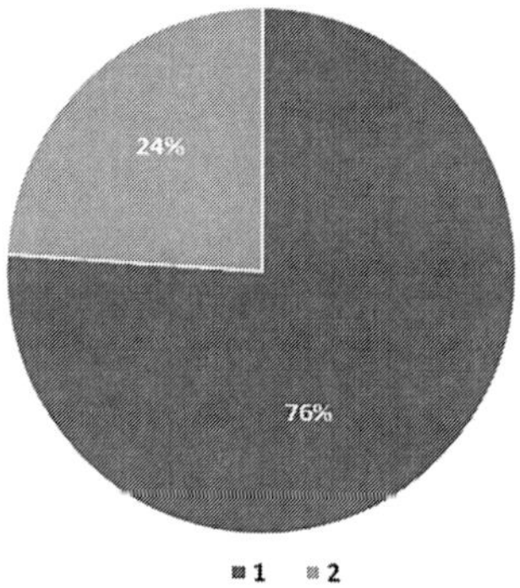

Minimum Spo2 : 35 (Rohidas Vithal Tankar)

Maximum HRCT : 20 (Yogesh Ramesh Mahashke)

Youngest : Sarthak Shelar (8 years)

Oldest : Sushila Jadhav (72years)

Patients with temperature > 102^{0}F: 9

Treatment protocol : 3 Step Flu Diet

Fan Therapy/ Prone Ventillation/ CAAT: 14

Cold Fomentation : 09

Medications: 0

Death: 0

Minimum recovery time: 4 days (51 patients)

Maximum recovery time: 7 days (21 patients)

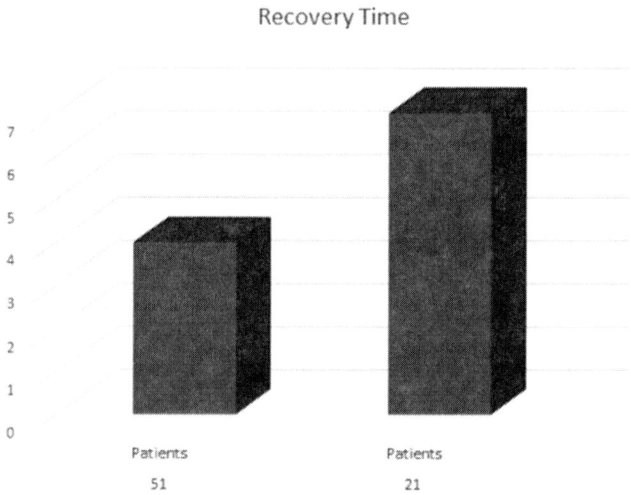
Recovery Time
7
6
5
4
3
2
1
0
Patients
51
Patients
21

25 Exclusive Stories

Fabiflu Complicated Health Condition

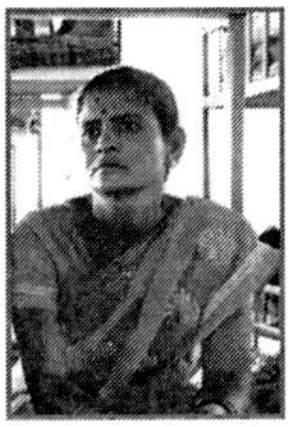

Medical History of the Patient before admission in N.I.C.E Centre:

Name: Rohini Walunj

Gender : Female **Age :** 39 years

Residence: Kaknewadi-Maharashtra.

Diagnosis: Covid-19, Fever, Weakness, Body ache

SpO2: 80

Hospitalised: No **Vaccinated :** No

Medications taken: Fabiflu

Status at the time of admission in N.I.C.E Centre

Date of Admission in N.I.C.E Centre: 25.05.2021

Date of Discharge: 03.06.2021

Discomforts: Fever 102°F /Weakness/Body Ache/Congestion/ Cough/Breathlessness. SPO2:80, HRCT Score: 7/25

Treatment Protocol/Intervention given in N.I.C.E Centre

1. 3-Step Flu Diet/ Raw Turmeric/Decoction
2. Cold Fomentation
3. Prone Ventilation

Medications: Nil

Outcome: After 7 days

Status: Completely recovered

Discomforts: Nil

Under Care of N.I.C.E Expert: Mr. Amit Shimpi

Rohini Walunj, a 39-year-old woman diagnosed with COVID 19, took heavy doses of allopathic medicines like Fabiflu. Her condition worsened, so she decided to get herself admitted to the N.I.C.E Centre, on 25th May 2021 with Covid-19 positive report, high fever, congestion, severe weakness and low oxygen saturation level of 80. Her HRCT score was 7/25.

She was assigned to N.I.C.E. expert Amit Shimpi who immediately put her on the 3-Step Flu Diet along with raw turmeric and decoction. She was given cold fomentation to lower down her body temperature.

She was put on prone ventilation position to increase her SpO2 levels. Within 24 hours by following the N.I.C.E protocol, her SpO2 level raised to 90, and third day onwards, it was above 95.

Describing the environment of Ahmednagar N.I.C.E Care Centre Rohini Walunj says, "The environment here is harmonious and amicable. I am happy to see the N.I.C.E experts and the caregivers without masks helping the patients with true love and compassion."

Watch her video testimonial at
www.coronakaal.tv/delta72

Vaccination transmitted Covid-19

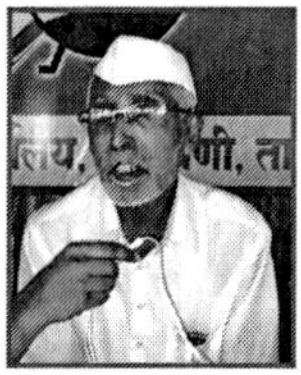

Medical History of the Patient before admission in N.I.C.E Centre:

Name: Vittal Fatty Hande, Age 65 years

Gender : Male

Residence: Bhojdari-.Maharashtra.

Diagnosis: Covid-19 positive, Fever, Weakness, Body ache

Hospitalised: No

Vaccination: Both doses of Covid-19 Vaccine

Medications taken: Nil

Status at the time of admission in N.I.C.E Centre

Date of Admission: 25.05.2021

Date of Discharge: 03.06.2021

Discomforts: Weakness&Body ache

Treatment Protocol/Intervention given in N.I.C.E Centre

1. 3 Step flu diet/Raw turmeric/decoction

Medications: Nil

Outcome: After 3 days

Status: Completely recovered

Discomforts: Nil

N.I.C.E Expert: Ms.Vaishnavi Walunj

A concerned 65-year-old farmer, Vittal Fatty Hande, was rushed to N.I.C.E Centre, on 25th May 2021, with symptoms like severe weakness and body ache. Because of taking both doses of the vaccine (on 13th March 2021 and 15th May 2021), he became Covid-19 positive.

He was scared to death but considered himself fortunate, that he was taken care of by N.I.C.E expert Vaishnavi Walunj.

He was given 3-Step Flu Diet along with raw turmeric and decoction. Within 24hrs he started feeling better and in 3 days, he completely recovered. He was so happy with the results of the 3-Step Flu Diet that he chose not to consume cooked food (though allowed to have cooked food once a day) so that he can detoxify himself.

He was happy to see the togetherness, love, compassion, and "Mask Free Zone" in the N.I.C.E Centre.

He is thankful to Dr.Biswaroop Roy Chowdhury and Mr. Nilesh Lanke for their philanthropic work. He has decided to educate people about not taking the Covid-19 vaccine.

Watch his video testimonial at
www.coronakaal.tv/delta72

Animal Like Treatment in Hospital

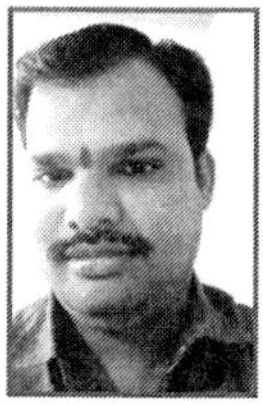

Medical History of the Patient before admission in N.I.C.E Centre:

Name: Yogesh Ramesh Mashke

Age: 33 years

Gender : Male

Residence: Navanagapur Dist- Ahmednagar

Diagnosis: Covid-19 positive, HRCT Score: 20/25, SPOR-70

Hospitalised: For 6 days in Daily Care Hospital in Ahmednagar

Vaccinated : No

Medications taken: Remdisivir Injection100mg, Saline solution,PAN Injection, EMSET 4mg Injection, Meropenom Injection, Targocid Injection, MPS 40 TDS Inhection, DOXY 100BD Injection, Sumol Stat Injection, SODABICARB STAT Injection, Hydrocort Stat Injection, Clexane Injection, Methylene Blue40 Injection, LevofloxIjnjection, Fabiflu Tablet

---

Status at the time of admission in N.I.C.E Centre

Date of Admission: 27.05.2021

Date of Discharge: 03.06.2021

Discomforts: Breathlessness, Weakness

Treatment Protocol/Intervention given in N.I.C.E Centre

1. 3 Step Flu Diet/
2. Prone ventilation and
3. Fan Therapy

Medications: Nil

Outcome: In 7 days

Status: Completely recovered

Discomforts: Nil

N.I.C.E Expert: Mr. Santosh Sarkale and Mr. Suresh V Garad

Covid -19 has shattered and broken many families including draining them financially. The story of Yogesh Ramesh Mashke, a 34-year-old labourer from a village in Ahmednagar Maharashtra, paints a picture of the countless lives which suffered due to Covid-19 pandemic in India.

Yogesh's ordeal began the moment he started having Covid-19 symptoms. As expected, he did the obvious thing and approached Daily Care Hospital in Ahmednagar. The hospital asked him to immediately deposit INR 60,000. He was forced to sell his motorbike, two mobile phones and his wife's gold chain to arrange the money.

As he got admitted, the hospital immediately started administering him with 4-5 bottles of saline per day along with 14 – 15 different tablets. To worsen the situation plethora of blood tests were conducted around his naval region, and each test costing him INR 8000. As the days progressed, so did his agony, as he started to run out of money.

On the 6th day, his physical condition deteriorated, and the hospital asked him to deposit more money for the treatment to continue. Unable to arrange for the money, Yogesh was forced to take discharge from the hospital.

Fortunately, he came in touch with N.I.C.E experts who got him admitted at the N.I.C. E Centre. At the time of admission into the N.I.C.E center, his HRCT Score was 20 and SpO2-70.

As per protocol he was immediately put in the prone position and the 3-Step Flu Diet started. Instead of medicines, he was administered, with love and compassion, two important pillars of the N.I.C.E protocol.

He got discharged within seven days after recovering fully.

“While I was in Daily Care Hospital, I was tied up with several tubes and felt like an animal. The moment I came under the treatment of N.I.C.E protocol, I began to feel much better. From second day onwards I was able to take five rounds around the N.I.C.E Centre. I feel blessed that I ran out of money and got discharged from the hospital and got the opportunity to get treated under the N.I.C.E protocol,” says Yogesh. Now a happy and healthy man, Yogesh gained the confidence and claims himself as a Corona Doctor and promises to treat people under the N.I.C.E protocol.

Watch his video testimonial at
www.coronakaal.tv/delta72

Love and Compassion cures Family of Three

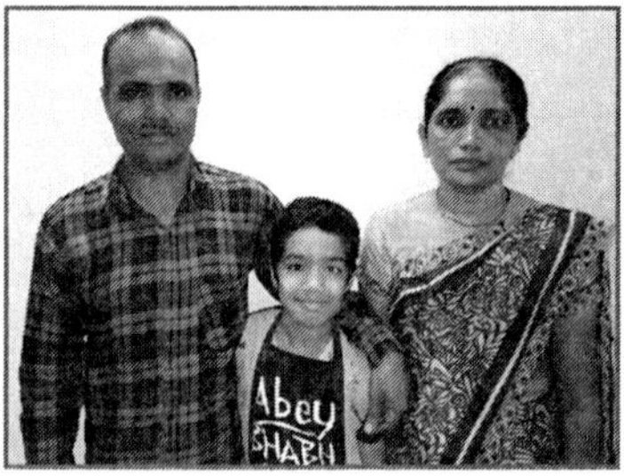

Medical History of the Patient before admission in N.I.C.E Centre:

Name: Sachin Shelar

Age: 42 years **Gender:** Male

Residence: Kedgaon-Maharashtra.

Diagnosis: Covid-19, Fever 101°F, Sore throat and Headache

Hospitalised: No **Vaccinated:** No

Medications taken: No

Status at the time of admission in N.I.C.E Centre

Date of Admission in N.I.C.E Centre: 30.05.2021

Date of Discharge: 03.06.2021

Discomforts: Fever 101°F, Sore throat and Headache

Treatment Protocol/Intervention given in N.I.C.E Centre

1. 3-Step Flu Diet/Raw turmeric/decoction

Medications: Nil

Outcome: After 4 days

Status: Completely recovered

Discomforts: Nil

Under Care of N.I.C.E Expert: Mr. Santosh Sarkale

Medical History of the Patient before admission in N.I.C.E Centre:

Name: KalpnaShelar

Age: 38 years, Gender-Female

Residence: Kedgaon-Maharashtra.

Diagnosis: Covid-19, Fever 100.5°F, Sore throat and Headache

Hospitalised: No

Vaccinated: No

Medications taken: Nil

Status at the time of admission in N.I.C.E Centre

Date of Admission in N.I.C.E Centre:30.05.2021

Date of Discharge: 03.06.2021

Discomforts: Sore throat and Headache

Treatment Protocol/Intervention given in N.I.C.E Centre

1. 3-Step Flu Diet/Raw turmeric/decoction

Medications: Nil

Outcome: After 4 days

Status: Completely recovered

Discomforts: Nil

Under Care of N.I.C.E Expert: Mr. Santosh Sarkale

Medical History of the Patient before admission in N.I.C.E Centre:

Name : Sarthak Shelar

Age: 8 years, Gender-Male

Residence: Kedgaon-Maharashtra.

Diagnosis: Covid-19, Fever 100°F and Sore throat

Hospitalised: No

Vaccinated: No

Medications taken: Nil

Status at the time of admission in N.I.C.E Centre

Date of Admission in N.I.C.E Centre: 30.05.2021

Date of Discharge: 03.06.2021

Discomforts: Fever 100°F and Sore throat

Treatment Protocol/Intervention given in N.I.C.E Centre

1. 3 Step Flu Diet/Raw turmeric/decoction

Medications: Nil

Outcome: After 4 days

Status: Completely recovered

Discomforts: Nil

Under Care of N.I.C.E Expert: Mr. Santosh Sarkale

Sachin Shelar, his wife Kalpana and son Sarthak got admitted to N.I.C.E Centre, on 30th May 2021, after being diagnosed as Covid-19 positive. They had symptoms such as Fever(100-101°F), sore throat and headache.

All of them were taken care of by N.I.C.E expert Santosh Sarkale, who immediately put them on the 3-Step Flu Diet along with raw turmeric and decoction.

The family was astonished and felt that they were residing in a "Mask Free Zone" and N.I.C.E experts were sitting next to them without maintaining any social distancing and most importantly, they got cured with 'Zero Medicine'.

The family recovered quickly, within four days and vowed that they will spread awareness about the Covid 19 treatment based on N.I.C.E protocol with 3-Step Flu Diet.

Watch their video testimonial at
www.coronakaal.tv/delta72

Family of Three Pledges Not To Wear Masks Ever Again

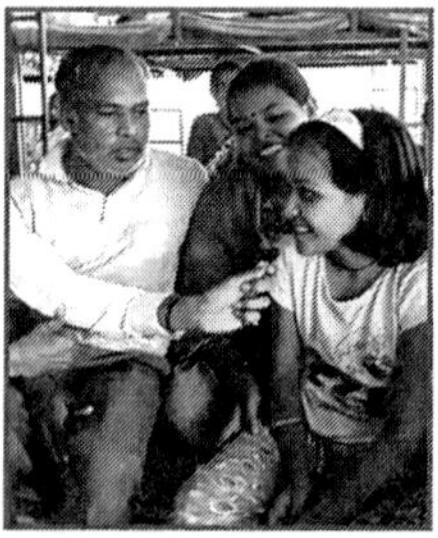

Medical History of the Patient before admission in N.I.C.E Centre:

Name: Avinash Kadam

Age:44 years, **Gender:** Male

Residence: Panoli-Maharashtra.

Diagnosis: Covid-19, Fever 104°F, Sore throat, Congestion, Breathlessness, HRCT score:11/25

Hospitalised: No **Vaccinated:** No

Medications taken: No

Status at the time of admission in N.I.C.E Centre

Date of Admission in N.I.C.E Centre: 25.05.2021

Date of Discharge: 03.06.2021

Discomforts: Fever 104°F, Sore throat, Congestion, Breathlessness, HRCT score:11/25

Treatment Protocol/Intervention given in N.I.C.E Centre

1. 3-Step Flu Diet/Raw turmeric/Decoction
2. Cold Fomentation

Medications: Nil

Outcome: After 7 days

Status: Completely recovered

Discomforts: NilUnder Care of N.I.C.E Expert: Mr. Amit Shimpi

---

Medical History of the Patient before admission in N.I.C.E Centre:

Name: Ujjwala A Kadam,

Age: 30 years, **Gender:** Female

Residence: Panoli-Maharashtra.

Diagnosis: Covid-19, Fever101°F, Weakness, Body Ache, Congestion

Hospitalised: No **Vaccinated:** No

Medications taken: Nil

Status at the time of admission in N.I.C.E Centre

Date of Admission in N.I.C.E Centre: 26.05.2021

Date of Discharge: 03.06.2021

Discomforts: Fever101°F, Weakness, Body Ache, Congestion

Treatment Protocol/Intervention given in N.I.C.E Centre

1. 3-Step Flu Diet/Raw turmeric/Decoction

Medications: Nil

Outcome: After 7 days

Status: Completely recovered

Discomforts: Nil

Under Care of N.I.C.E Expert: Mr. Amit Shimpi

Medical History of the Patient before admission in N.I.C.E Centre:

Name: ShravaniAvinash Kadam

Age: 10 years, **Gender:** Female

Residence: Panoli-Maharashtra.

Diagnosis: Covid-19, Fever 102°F, Weakness, Body Ache, Congestion & Cough

Hospitalised: No **Vaccinated:** No

Medications taken: Nil

Status at the time of admission in N.I.C.E Centre

Date of Admission in N.I.C.E Centre: 26.05.2021

Date of Discharge: 03.06.2021

Discomforts: Fever 102°F, Weakness, Body Ache, Congestion & Cough

---

Treatment Protocol/Intervention given in N.I.C.E Centre

1. 3-Step Flu Diet/Raw turmeric/Decoction
2. Cold fomentation

Medications:Nil

Outcome: After 5 days

Status: Completely recovered

Discomforts: Nil

Under Care of N.I.C.E Expert: Mr. Amit Shimpi

Avinash Kadam, a resident of Panoli Maharashtra, was detected as Covid-19 positive on May 2021. The ordeal and the long struggle just began. As soon as he tested positive, his wife Ujjwala and 10-year-old daughter Shravani too tested positive. A barber by profession, Covid-19 hit them hard where it hurts the most - on their pockets. Initially, they were clueless and didn't know what to do. Then an acquaintance gave them the suggestion to get in touch at N.I.C.E Centre. They got in touch with the N.I.C.E team on 25th May 2021 and got admitted the next day at N.I.C.E Centre.

Avinash struggled with fever as high as 104 °F, Ujjwala 101 °F and Shravani102 °F, they were immediately put on the 3-Step Flu Diet. Avinash and his daughter were given cold fomentation to bring down the high fever. Additional protocols for chest congestion and headache were also followed for his wife and daughter.

On the fourth day, around 3.30 am Shravani developed loose motions and became restless, constantly demanding medicine. However, as per N.I.C.E treatment protocol, the N.I.C.E experts put her on '3-Step Stomach Protocol' following which, Shravani recovered by afternoon.

Avinash talking about his recovery journey says, "I feel good without consuming any medicines. I am so happy that just based on a diet of fruits and coconut water, I have completely recovered."

Sharing her experience, Ujwalla says, "I was under a lot of pain when I reached here. I was constantly coughing and also had high fever. I started feeling much better after having the ginger decoction and fruits. Next time if any one of us falls sick, we will follow the 3-Step Flu Diet to cure ourselves. And importantly, we will no longer wear masks, as it becomes difficult to breathe while wearing one."

The family recovered within seven days and walked out of the Covid-19 Center with smiles and joy in their hearts.

Watch their video testimonial at www.coronakaal.tv/delta72

Vaccination Proves Fatal for the Sister Duo

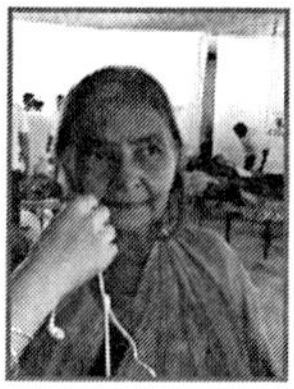

Medical History of the Patient before admission in N.I.C.E Centre:

Name: Babaee Vilas kanade **Age:** 61 years

Gender : Female

Residence: Devdaitan-Junnar, Pune-Maharashtra

Diagnosis: Fever/Chest Congestion/ Cough/ Headache

Hospitalised: No

Vaccination: took the first dose of Covid-19 vaccine

Medications taken: No

Status at the time of admission in N.I.C.E Centre

Date of Admission: 25.05.2021

Date of Discharge: 03.06.2021

Discomforts: Breathlessness, Weakness

Treatment Protocol/Intervention given in N.I.C.E Centre

1. 3-Step Flu Diet, Raw Turmeric and Decoction

Medications: Nil

Outcome: In 7 days

Status: Completely recovered

Discomforts: Nil

N.I.C.E Expert: Ms. Chitra Jain

Medical History of the Patient before admission in N.I.C.E Centre:

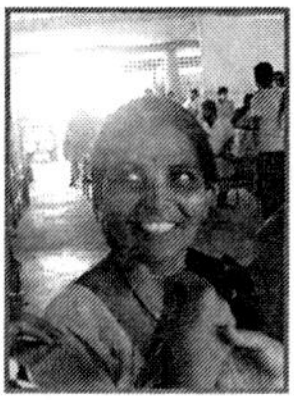

Name: Manisha Kaluram kadam

Age: 40 years **Gender :** Female

Residence: Devdaitan-Junnar, Pune-Maharashtra

Diagnosis: Chest Congestion/ Cough/Ribs pain

Hospitalised: No **Vaccination:** No

Medications taken: No

Status at the time of admission in N.I.C.E Centre

Date of Admission: 25.05.2021

Date of Discharge: 03.06.2021

Discomforts: Chest Congestion/ Cough/Ribs pain

Treatment Protocol/Intervention given in N.I.C.E Centre

1. 3-Step Flu Diet, Raw Turmeric and Decoction

Medications: Nil

Outcome: In 7 days

Status: Completely recovered

Discomforts: Nil

N.I.C.E Expert: Ms. Chitra Jain

Babee Vilas Kanade and Manisha Kaluram Kadam, both the sisters, could hardly imagine that in 2021, they would have to witness pain and agony. 61-year-old Babaee followed the popular belief of safeguarding oneself from the Covid-19 virus and she got herself vaccinated with the first dose. Little did she know that the vaccine, instead of saving her life could prove fatal.

Immediately after taking the vaccine, she developed Covid-19 symptoms, like high fever, chest congestion and headache for consecutively 15 days. Meanwhile Babee further transmitted infection to her sister Manisha who developed Covid-19 symptoms like chest congestion, cough and severe rib pain.

After bearing the ordeal for odd 15 days, she got herself admitted to N.I.C.E Centre, along with her sister.

N.I.C.E expert Chitra Jain started monitoring both the sisters and promptly started the 3-Step Flu Diet coupled with raw turmeric and the standard decoction. Both the sisters recovered within six days and got discharged.

Talking about her experience, Babee Vilas says, "It was my mistake to get vaccinated. After what I have gone through, I have decided not to get my second dose. We consider ourselves lucky that we got treated under the N.I.C.E protocol, which saved our lives."

Watch their video testimonial at
www.coronakaal.tv/delta72

SpO2-35,Temkar becomes Suicidal and Slips into Depression

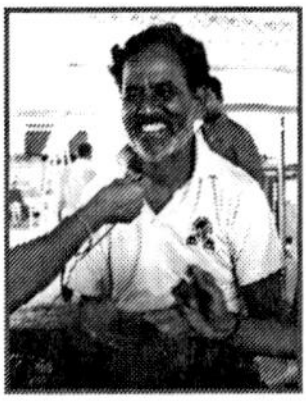

Medical History of the Patient before admission in N.I.C.E Centre:

Name: Temkar Rohidas Vitthal

Age: 45 years, **Gender:** Male

Residence: Pimparkhed -Maharashtra.

Diagnosis: Covid 19, Breathing difficulty, Weakness

Hospitalised: Allopathic ward of Covid Centre

Vaccinated: No

Medications taken: Fabiflu

Status at the time of admission in N.I.C.E Centre

Date of Admission in N.I.C.E Centre: 27.05.2021

Date of Discharge: 03.06.2021

Discomforts: Weakness, Breathing difficulty, SpO2-35

Treatment Protocol/Intervention given in N.I.C.E Centre

1. 3-Step Flu Diet/Raw turmeric/decoction
2. Prone Ventilation/fan theraphy

Medications: Nil

Outcome: After 5 days

Status: Completely recovered

Discomforts: Nil

Under Care of N.I.C.E Experts: Mr. Amit Shimpi, Ms.Vaishnavi Walunj, Ms. Chitra Jain, Mr. Avinash Sabare

When Temkar Rohidas Vitthal, a 45-year-old farmer, was diagnosed as Covid-19 positive, his family members disowned him with the fear that they too might get infected. He was sent to a COVID Centre and was administered with heavy doses of medication such as Fabiflu, but instead of getting better, his condition worsened. From a normal SpO2 level his oxygen saturation dropped to 35. This shattered him mentally and he started having suicidal thoughts and slipped into depression. On 27th May 2021, he decided to shift to the N.I.C.E Centre.

N.I.C.E experts Vaishnavi Walunj, Amit Shimpi and Avinash Popatrao took up the challenge to cure him. They not only started his treatment as per N.I.C.E Protocol but also counselled and motivated him.

He was given the 3-Step Flu Diet, raw turmeric, decoction and was put in prone ventilation position. Steadily his saturation level (SpO2) started to increase and reached 77. From here N.I.C.E expert Chitra Jain took over.

The 3-Step Fu Diet was continued, along with prone ventilation and fan therapy.

On the fifth day, his SpO2 level was 91 and after a couple of days, the reading went up to 98.

A happy man, ready to accept the challenge to run around the N.I.C.E Centre and changing his surname from Temkar to Lanke as a mark of gratitude to Mr. Nilesh Lanke (MLA Ahmednagar) who saved his life. He went home safe and sound!

Watch his video testimonial at www.coronakaal.tv/delta72

65-year-old Comorbid Patient Recovered in 4 Days

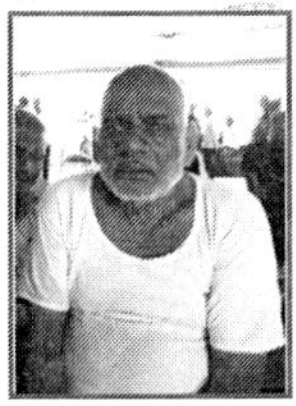

Medical History of the Patient before admission in N.I.C.E Centre:

Name: Ramesh Buchude

Age: 65 years, **Gender:** Male

Residence: Baburdi Village, Parner-Maharashtra.

Diagnosis: Covid-19, Fever 105°F, Weakness, Body

Ache, Headache, Sore throat, SpO2 : 85

Hospitalised: No **Vaccinated:** No

Medications taken: Nil

Status at the time of admission in N.I.C.E Centre

Date of Admission in N.I.C.E Centre: 29.05.2021

Date of Discharge: 03.06.2021

Discomforts: Fever 105°F, Weakness, Body Ache, Headache, Sore throat, SpO2 : 85

Treatment Protocol/Intervention given in N.I.C.E Centre

1. 3-Step Flu Diet/Raw Turmeric/Decoction
2. Cold Fomentation
3. Prone Ventilation

Medications: Nil

Outcome: After 4 days

Status: Completely recovered

Discomforts: Nil

Under Care of N.I.C.E Expert: Mr. Prateek Joshi

Ramesh Buchude, a 65-year-old diabetic person, got diagnosed, Covid-19 positive and got admitted to N.I.C.E Centre, on 29th May 2021, with severe symptoms such as breathlessness, low SpO2 level at 85, fever as high as 105°F.

N.I.C.E expert Prateek Joshi took good care of him and immediately put him on the 3-Step Flu Diet, along with raw turmeric and decoction. He was given cold fomentation to lower down his fever and was made to lie in prone position so that his SpO2 level can increase.

With N.I.C.E experts love care & motivation, Ramesh, with comorbidities & severe symptoms, recovered quickly within four days.

He gives the credit of his recovery to the Mask-Free environment of the N.I.C.E Centre and to the 3-Step Flu Diet plan.

Watch his video testimonial at
www.coronakaal.tv/delta72

HRCT-19/25 Driver takes a U-turn from Hospital Death Bed to a Healthy Jumping Jack

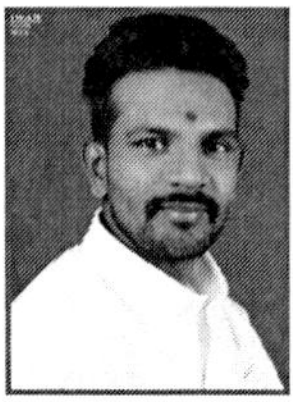

Medical History of the Patient before admission in N.I.C.E Centre:

Name: Nilesh Ghumatkar, **Age:** 24 years,
Gender: Male
Residence: Parner-Maharashtra.
Diagnosis: Covid-19, Fever 102.5°F, Body ache,Weakness, Chest congestion, Severe cough,Breathlessness, HRCT:19/25, SpO2-90
Hospitalized: Yes **Vaccinated:** No
Medications taken: Fabiflu, Saline solution

Status at the time of admission in N.I.C.E Centre

Date of Admission in N.I.C.E Centre: 30.05.2021
Date of Discharge: 03.06.2021
Discomforts: Fever 102°F, Body ache, Headache, Weakness, Chest congestion, Severe cough, Breathlessness, HRCT:19/25, SpO2-90

Treatment Protocol/Intervention given in N.I.C.E Centre

1. 3-Step Flu Diet/Raw Turmeric/Decoction
2. Cold Fomentation
3. Prone Ventilation

Medications: Nil
Outcome: After 4 days

Status: Completely recovered
Discomforts: Nil
Under Care of N.I.C.E Experts: Mr. Santosh, Sarkale, Mr. Avinash Popatrao Sabare & Ms. Seema Mannikoth

Nilesh Ghumatkar, a 24-year-old man, working as a driver with MLA Nilesh Lanke, made the biggest mistake of his life by getting himself admitted to a private hospital in Parner district Maharashtra, once he was detected Covid-19 positive. At the time of admission into the hospital, he was under the moderate category, but due to hospital interventions (Fabiflu along with 16 other medicines three times a day), his condition became severe. He was also administered seven bottles of saline per day. After five days of undergoing treatment at the hospital and having near to death experience, at the advice of his boss, MLA Nilesh Lanke, he got admitted to N.I.C.E Centre.

He came to the N.I.C.E Centre with an extremely deteriorated health condition with fever 102°F and an HRCT Score of 19/25, along with severe body ache, weakness, headache and chest congestion.
His treatment started under the N.I.C.E protocol and his health condition took a complete U-Turn. By the third day, he started to walk around the N.I.C.E Centre. On the fourth day, he felt much better and sported a big smile on his face.
Talking about his recovery journey, Nilesh says, "I am returning as a happy and a healthy man, follower of DIP Diet & quitting non-vegetarian food."
What a U-turn...!

Watch his video testimonial at www.coronakaal.tv/delta72

Pregnant Woman N.I.C.E(ly) Cured

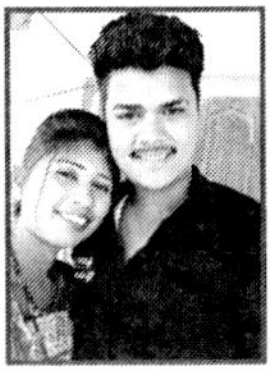

Medical History of the Patient before admission in N.I.C.E Centre:

Name : Ashok Manchare,

Age: 21years, male

Residence: Tikhol -Maharashtra.

Diagnosis: Covid-19, Fever 102°F /Weakness/Body Ache/Congestion.

Hospitalised: No **Vaccinated:** No

Medications taken: Nil

Status at the time of admission in N.I.C.E Centre

Date of Admission in N.I.C.E Centre: 25.05.2021

Date of Discharge: 03.06.2021

Discomforts: Fever 102°F /Weakness/Body Ache/Congestion.

Treatment Protocol/Intervention given in N.I.C.E Centre

1. 3-Step Flu Diet/Raw Turmeric/Decoction
2. Cold Fomentation

Medications: Nil

Outcome: After 7 days

Status: Completely recovered

Discomforts: Nil

Under Care of N.I.C.E Expert: Mr. Amit Shimpi

Medical History of the Patient before admission in N.I.C.E Centre:

Name: Kajal Ashok Manchare(5 Month Pregnant).

Age: 20years , female

Residence: Tikhol -Maharashtra.

Diagnosis: Covid-19, Fever 103°F /Weakness/Body Ache

Hospitalised: No **Vaccinated:** No

Medications taken: Nil

Status at the time of admission in N.I.C.E Centre

Date of Admission in N.I.C.E Centre: 27.05.2021

Date of Discharge: 03.06.2021

Discomforts: Fever 103°F /Weakness/Body Ache

Treatment Protocol/Intervention given in N.I.C.E Centre

1. 3-Step Flu Diet/Raw Turmeric/Decoction
2. Cold Fomentation

Medications: Nil

Outcome: After 5 days

Status: Completely recovered

Discomforts: Nil

Under Care of N.I.C.E Expert: Mr. Amit Shimpi and Ms. Seema Mannikoth.

Young couple Ashok Manchare and his five months pregnant wife Kajal Manchare, from Tikol Maharashtra, together fought

Covid-19 with flying colours. 21-year-old farmer Ashok got admitted to N.I.C.E Centre, with 102°F fever.

Ashok also had weakness and body ache; he was immediately assigned to N.I.C.E expert Dr. Amit Shimpi. He was given the 3-Step Flu Diet along with other remedies. As he was on his path to recovery, he discovered that his 19-year-old wife, too was a Covid-19 positive with a fever of 103°F; he immediately advised Kajal to join him at the N.I.C.E Centre. As she was five months pregnant, the couple's concern was, since they have to be on zero medicines, how Kajal would receive her required folic acid and vitamins, which she to date was deriving from allopathic medicines. The N.I.C.E experts patiently educated them on the drawbacks of the allopathic medicines and made them aware of the health benefits of various kinds of vegetable juices, nut milk and coconut water.

The couple understood the importance of deriving health benefits from fruits and vegetables as source of nutrition and not mindlessly consuming allopathic medicines. Kajal was then given the 3-Step Flu Diet and other remedies under the N.I.C. E protocol.

Both recovered within five days. Talking about his experience, Ashok says, "We are happy and also feel healthy. What we appreciate the most; is that neither the caregivers nor any of the patients were allowed to wear masks. The environment was of true love and compassion that helps the patients to heal faster. We give our heartfelt gratitude to Dr. Biswaroop Roy Chowdhury and Mr. Nilesh Lanke for their humanitarian work."

The empathy and kindness of the N.I.C.E experts touched Ashok so much that, after his recovery, he volunteered and helped the patients who were admitted in the N.I.C.E Centre.

The couple went back fully recovered with a heart full of gratitude and nutritional knowledge to take care of themselves and their future generation.

Watch their video testimonial at
www.coronakaal.tv/delta72

Suffering from Adverse Effects of Vaccination

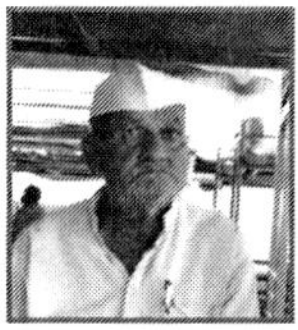

Medical History of the Patient before admission in N.I.C.E Centre:

Name: Bhivsen Ghadge **Age**: 69 years

Gender: Male,

Residence: Nimgaon Sava Tal, Junnar Distt, Pune-Maharashtra.

Diagnosis: Dry cough and weakness

Hospitalised: No **Vaccination:** (First dose of Covid-19 Vaccine)

Medications taken: Nil

Status at the time of admission in N.I.C.E Centre

Date of Admission: 25.05.2021

Date of Discharge: 03.06.2021

Discomforts: Dry cough and weakness

Treatment Protocol/Intervention given in N.I.C.E Centre

1. 3-Step Flu Diet
2. Raw turmeric
3. Decoction

Medications: Nil

Outcome: After 4days

Status: Completely recovered

Discomforts: Nil

N.I.C.E Expert: Mr. Santosh Sarkale

Bhivsen Ghadge, a 69-year-old man, got himself vaccinated with the first dose of the Covid-19 vaccine on 1stApril 2021 and soon developed Covid-19 symptoms such as severe cough and weakness.

On 25th May 2021, on the advice of one of his relatives, he got himself admitted to N.I.C.E Centre. Though he stays 100 km away from the centre, he got himself admitted.

N.I.C.E expert Mr. Santosh Sarkale started monitoring him and gave him the 3-Step Flu Diet coupled with raw turmeric and decoction. He recovered within four days.

Talking about his experience, Bhivsen Ghadge says, "It was not a good decision to get vaccinated." After his experience with the N.I.C.E protocol, he has decided not to consume any food item derived from animals, especially dairy products. He considers himself fortunate that he got himself treated under the N.I.C.E protocol.

Watch his video testimonial at
www.coronakaal.tv/delta72

10-Month Old Toddler joins in to support Covid 19 father

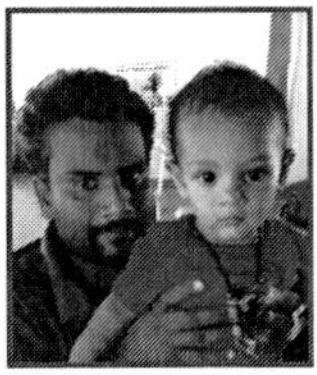

Medical History of the Patient before admission in N.I.C.E Centre:

Name: Kripashankar Yadav, **Age:** 34 years

Gender : Male

Residence: Ahmednagar-Maharashtra.

Diagnosis: Covid-19 with Fever 102°F /Weakness/ Congestion/ SpO2: 87

Hospitalised: No **Vaccinated:** No

Medications taken: Nil

Status at the time of admission in N.I.C.E Centre

Date of Admission in N.I.C.E Centre: 26.05.2021

Date of Discharge: 03.06.2021

Discomforts: Fever 102°F /Weakness/ Congestion/ Cough/ Breathlessness. SpO2:87

Treatment Protocol/Intervention given in N.I.C.E Centre

1 3-Step Flu Diet/Raw Turmeric/Decoction

2. Cold Fomentation

3. Prone Ventilation

Medications: Nil

Outcome: After 5 days
Status: Completely recovered
Discomforts: Nil
Under Care of N.I.C.E Expert: Ms. Chitra Jain

Kripa Shankar Yadav, a 34-year-old man, got admitted to the N.I.C.E Centre on 26thMay 2021, with a Covid-19 positive report, high fever, congestion and low oxygen level at 87.

He was assigned to N.I.C.E. expert Chitra Jain. He was given a 3-Step Flu Diet, along with decoction and raw turmeric. He was given cold fomentation to decrease his body temperature and made to lie down in a prone position, along with fan therapy, to improve his oxygen level. He started recovering slowly, but when his wife and 10-month-old son joined him in the N.I.C.E Centre, his recovery rate accelerated much faster. Toddler Rishab was a joyous addition to the N.I.C.E Centre, as he quickly became friendly and playful with all patients.

N.I.C.E. experts Chitra Jain and Seema Mannikkoth educated Kripa Shankar about health benefits of various kinds of fruits and coconut water main ingredients of the 3-Step Flu Diet. He recovered within five days.

Talking about his experience, Kripa Shankar says, "I found the environment very congenial and amicable. Without wearing masks, all N.I.C.E experts and caregivers were helping the patients with true love and compassion. I will spread the goodness and positive experience with others. I thank Dr. Biswaroop Roy Chowdhury and Mr. Nilesh Lanke, from the bottom of my heart, for their humanitarian work."

He was discharged on 3rd June 2021, fully recovered with a heart full of happiness and nutritional knowledge to take care of his family and the future generation.

Watch his video testimonial at www.coronakaal.tv/delta72

When Vaccination brought misery and agony to the entire family

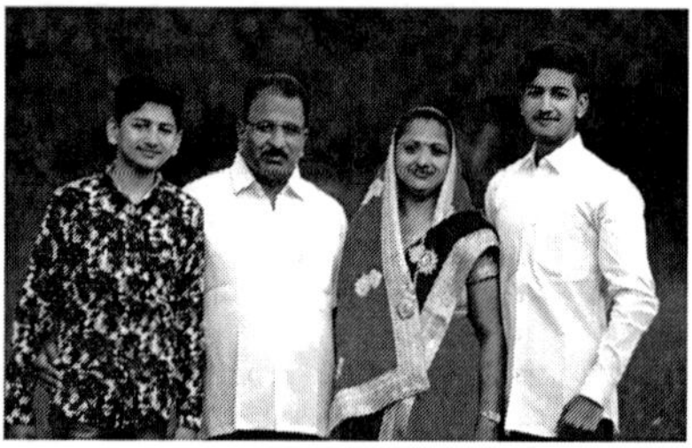

Medical History of the Patient before admission in N.I.C.E Centre:

Name: Prakash BankatlalMunot

Age: 52 years, **Gender:** Male

Residence: Kada Village Ashti Taluka -Maharashtra.

Diagnosis: Covid 19, Fever 99.5 °F /Weakness/Body Ache/ Congestion, SpO2:75

Hospitalised: Yes **Vaccinated:** Yes, first dose

Medications taken: Favimax400, Zostum1.5mg, Lomocare40mg, Prestirod40mg, Saline Solution

---

Status at the time of admission in N.I.C.E Centre

Date of Admission in N.I.C.E Centre: 25.05.2021

Date of Discharge: 03.06.2021

Discomforts: Fever 99.5°F /Weakness/Body Ache/SpO2-75.

Treatment Protocol/Intervention given in N.I.C.E Centre

1. 3 Step flu diet/Raw turmeric/decoction
2. Prone ventilation

Medications: Nil

Outcome: After 7 days

Status: Completely recovered

Discomforts: Nil

Under Care of N.I.C.E Expert: Ms. Vaishnavi Walunj

Medical History of the Patient before admission in N.I.C.E Centre:

Name: Sarika Munot

Age: 38 years, **Gender:** Female

Residence: Kada Village Ashti Taluka -Maharashtra.

Diagnosis: Covid 19, Sore throat and Headache

Hospitalised: No **Vaccinated:** No

Medications taken: Nil

Status at the time of admission in N.I.C.E Centre

Date of Admission in N.I.C.E Centre: 25.05.2021

Date of Discharge: 03.06.2021

Discomforts: Sore throat and Headache

Treatment Protocol/Intervention given in N.I.C.E Centre

1. 3 Step flu diet/Raw turmeric/decoction

Medications: Nil

Outcome: After 4 days

Status: Completely recovered

Discomforts: Nil

Under Care of N.I.C.E Expert: Mr. Santosh Sarkale

Medical History of the Patient before admission in N.I.C.E Centre:

Name: Mahavir Munot

Age: 19 years, **Gender:** Male

Residence: Kada Village Ashti Taluka -Maharashtra.

Diagnosis: Covid 19, Fever 101°F and Cough

Hospitalised: No **Vaccinated:** No

Medications taken: Nil

Status at the time of admission in N.I.C.E Centre

Date of Admission in N.I.C.E Centre: 25.05.2021

Date of Discharge: 03.06.2021

Discomforts: Fever 101°F and Cough

Treatment Protocol/Intervention given in N.I.C.E Centre

1. 3 Step flu diet/Raw turmeric/decoction

Medications: Nil

Outcome: After 4 days

Status: Completely recovered

Discomforts: Nil

Under Care of N.I.C.E Expert: Mr. Santosh Sarkale

Medical History of the Patient before admission in N.I.C.E Centre:

Name: Hardik Munot

Age: 15 years, **Gender:** Male

Residence: Kada Village Ashti Taluka -Maharashtra.

Diagnosis: Covid 19, Asymptomatic

Hospitalised: No **Vaccinated:** No

Medications taken: Nil

Status at the time of admission in N.I.C.E Centre

Date of Admission in N.I.C.E Centre: 25.05.2021

Date of Discharge: 03.06.2021

Discomforts: No discomfort

Treatment Protocol/Intervention given in N.I.C.E Centre

1. 3 Step flu diet/Raw turmeric/decoction

Medications: Nil

Outcome: After 4 days

Status: Completely recovered

Discomforts: Nil

Under Care of N.I.C.E Expert: Ms. Vaishnavi Walunj

Prakash Munot, a 52-year-old man from Kadahasti Maharashtra, took the first dose of the Covid-19 vaccine in April 2021, and soon developed symptoms of Covid-19. To make the situation worse he became the source of transmission of Covid-19 and infected his wife and both sons. Prakash did what the common belief is, to get oneself admitted to the hospital. In the hospital, he underwent numerous treatments, along with a plethora of allopathic medicines, like Favimax 400, Zostum, Lomocare, Prestirod along with continuous saline drips. Yet after five long days and a hefty bill of INR 60,000, his health kept on deteriorating. That's when Prakash decided to shift to the N.I.C.E Centre along with his wife and two sons.

When he got admitted to the N.I.C.E Centre, his SpO2 level was as low as 75 and he experienced severe weakness and body ache, and that's when N.I.C.E expert Vaishnavi Walunj took him under her care. The 3-Step Flu Diet, raw turmeric, decoction, prone ventilation with fan therapy was initiated immediately.

His wife Sarika, a 38-year-old housewife, had symptoms such as headache and weakness. The elder son, Mahavir Munot, a 19-year-old, had a fever and cough. He was put under care of N.I.C.E expert Santosh Sarkale. Younger son Hardik Munot, a 15-year-old boy, was Covid-19 positive & asymptomatic. He was put under the care of N.I.C.E expert Vaishnavi Walnuj.

As per N.I.C.E protocol 3 step Flu Diet was initiated for all of them

Family started to recover quickly giving credit to family like ambience in the N.I.C.E Centre. "While I was here, it always felt like home. I feel fortunate that I made the decision against allopathic treatment and instead came here. I am happy that my family also recovered quickly" says the father.

The family gives credit to the love & compassion of N.I.C.E. experts. They were happy to see that instead of social distancing, love and social gathering are curing people. Not only this, the entire family learned the N.I.C.E treatment Protocol so that they can guide and cure other people suffering from Covid-19.

The family walked out of the N.I.C.E Centre fully cured taking home a message of love, care, compassion and understanding the sham and irrelevance of masks and social distancing.

Watch their video testimonial at
www.coronakaal.tv/delta72

Fabiflu Fails for Saas-Bahu

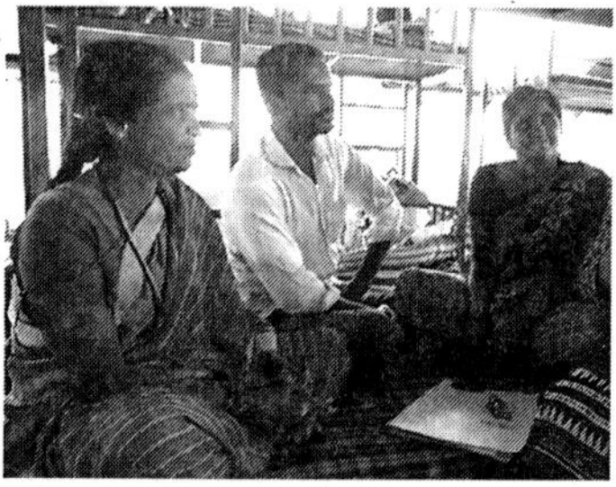

Medical History of the Patient before admission in N.I.C.E Centre:

Name: Nandkishor Dhokchulae

Age: 35 years, **Gender:** Male

Residence:-Shrirampur-Maharashtra.

Diagnosis: Covid-19,chest congestion and cough

Hospitalised: No **Vaccinated:** No

Medications taken: No

Status at the time of admission in N.I.C.E Centre

Date of Admission in N.I.C.E Centre: 25.05.2021

Date of Discharge: 03.06.2021

Discomforts: Chest congestion and Sore throat

Treatment Protocol/Intervention given in N.I.C.E Centre

1. 3-Step Flu Diet/Raw turmeric/decoction

Medications: Nil

Outcome: After 4days

Status: Completely recovered

Discomforts: Nil

Under Care of N.I.C.E Expert: Ms. Chitra Jain

Medical History of the Patient before admission in N.I.C.E Centre:

Name – Sita Bai Dhokchulae

Age- 50 years, Gender-Female

Residence: Shrirampur-Maharashtra.

Diagnosis: Covid-19, chest congestion and cough

Hospitalised: Zawarae Covid-19 Centre

Vaccinated: No

Medications taken: Fabiflu

Status at the time of admission in N.I.C.E Centre

Date of Admission in N.I.C.E Centre:25.05.2021

Date of Discharge: 03.06.2021

Discomforts: Sore throat and chest congestion

Treatment Protocol/Intervention given in N.I.C.E Centre

1. 3-Step Flu Diet/Raw turmeric/decoction

Medications:Nil

Outcome: After 4 days

Status: Completely recovered

Discomforts: Nil

Under Care of N.I.C.E Expert: Ms. Chitra Jain

Medical History of the Patient before admission in N.I.C.E Centre:

Name: Manisha Dhokchulae

Age: 32 years, **Gender:** Female

Residence: Shrirampur-Maharashtra.

Diagnosis: Covid positive, chest congestion and sore throat

Hospitalised: Zawarae Covid-19 Centre

Vaccinated: No

Medications taken: Fabiflu

Status at the time of admission in N.I.C.E Centre

Date of Admission in N.I.C.E Centre: 25.05.2021

Date of Discharge: 03.06.2021

Discomforts: Chest congestion and Sore throat

Treatment Protocol/Intervention given in N.I.C.E Centre

1. 3 Step Flu Diet/Raw turmeric/decoction

Medications: Nil

Outcome: After 4 days

Status: Completely recovered

Discomforts: Nil

Under Care of N.I.C.E Expert: Ms. Chitra Jain

Family of three Sita Bai (Mother) 50-year-old, Nandkishor Dokchulae (Son) 35-year-old and Manisha Dokchulae (Daughter-in-Law) 32- year-old, from Shrirampur, Maharashtra was suffering from chest congestion, cough, body ache and were Covid-19 positive.

Sita Bai and Manisha got themselves admitted to Zawarae Covid-19 Centre and were administered Fabiflu. Even after five days there was no relief. A family acquaintance advised them to get admitted to the N.I.C.E Centre.

A couple of hours away from their home, all three of them got admitted on 25th May 2021. Under the guidance of N.I.C.E. expert Chitra Jain, they all followed the 3-Step Flu Diet. They recovered within four days without any medicine.

Amazed, they credited their health recovery to the N.I.C.E protocol of 'No Mask' and 'No Medicine' and to the experts who took care of all the patients with love and empathy without social distancing.

Watch their video testimonial at www.coronakaal.tv/delta72

Other Patients' Seamless Recovery Through N.I.C.E Protocol

Patient **Kamal Govardhan Nimsae** from **Ahmednagar**, **Ahmednagar** age **52 years** yrs, **Female,** was admitted in N.I.C.E Centre on **26.05.2021** with the symptoms of **Fever 101°F/Weakness/Body Ache** got cured following 3 Step Flu Diet in **4 days** under the N.I.C.E care of **Chitra Jain**. After recovering completely, the patient was discharged on **03.06.2021**

Patient **Mahesh Madho Tajwe** from **Junner**, **Pune** age **24 yrs** yrs, **Male,** was admitted in N.I.C.E Centre on **25.05.2021** with the symptoms of **Fever/Chest Congestion/ Cough/Breathlessness, HRCT Score: 11/25** got cured following 3 Step Flu Diet in **4 days** under the N.I.C.E care of **Chitra Jain**. After recovering completely, the patient was discharged on **03.06.2021**

Patient **Sanjay prahlad Gangurde** from **Rahata**, **Ahmednagar** age **43 years** yrs, **Male,** was admitted in N.I.C.E Centre on **26.05.2021** with the symptoms of **Fever 101.7°F/Weakness:, HRCT:17/25** got cured following 3 Step Flu Diet in **4 days** under the N.I.C.E care of **Chitra Jain**. After recovering completely, the patient was discharged on **03.06.2021**

Patient **Dilip Shankar Lokhare** from **Nighoj**, **Parner** age **49** yrs, **Male,** was admitted in N.I.C.E Centre on **25.05.2021** with the symptoms of **Fever 103^{0}F/Congestion/cough, HRCT score:14/25** got cured following 3 Step Flu Diet in **5 to 7 days** under the N.I.C.E care of **Chitra Jain**. After recovering completely, the patient was discharged on **03.06.2021**

Patient **Sunita Sayyaji Shelar** from **Belwandi. Shrigonda**, **Ahmednagar** age **45** yrs, **Female,** was admitted in N.I.C.E Centre on **27.05.2021** with the symptoms of **Fever102°F, Breathing difficulty, SPO2 86-90, HRCT Score-15/25** got cured following 3 Step Flu Diet in **5 to 7 days** under the N.I.C.E care of **Chitra Jain**. After recovering completely, the patient was discharged on **09.06.2021**

Patient **Walmik B. Kolhe** from **Loni Haveli**, **Loni Haveli** age **37** yrs, **Male,** was admitted in N.I.C.E Centre on **25.05.2021** with the symptoms of **Fever102°F /Weakness/Body Ache/Congestion** got cured following 3 Step Flu Diet in **4 days** under the N.I.C.E care of **Amit Shimpi**. After recovering completely, the patient was discharged on **03.06.2021**

Patient **Asif Najar Shiekh** from **Bella**, **Bella** age **34** yrs, **Male,** was admitted in N.I.C.E Centre on **29.05.2021** with the symptoms of **Fever102°F/Breathlessness/Weakness SPO2:58** got cured following 3 Step Flu Diet in **4** under the N.I.C.E care of **Prateek Joshi**. After recovering completely, the patient was discharged on

---

Patient **Avinash Ramnath Kharat** from **Otur**, **OTUR** age **27** yrs, **Male,** was admitted in N.I.C.E Centre on **30.05.2021** with the symptoms of **Sore throat/Congestion/Cough/Headache/Weakness, HRCT Score:4/25** got cured following 3 Step Flu Diet in **4 days** under the N.I.C.E care of **Prateek Joshi**. After recovering completely, the patient was discharged on **03.06.2021**

Patient **Chandrakant Rokade** from **A/P Kharjule Harya Tal- Parner Dist- Ahmednagar**, **Kharjule Harya** age **53 yrs** yrs, **Male,** was admitted in N.I.C.E Centre on **25.05.2021** with the symptoms of **Dry cough, bodyache, breathlessness, SPO2 89** got cured following 3 Step Flu Diet in **4 days** under the N.I.C.E care of **Santosh Sarkale**. After recovering completely, the patient was discharged on **03.06.2021**

Patient **Ishwar Gangrade** from **batodi gaon**, **batodi** age **50** yrs, **Male,** was admitted in N.I.C.E Centre on

30.05.2021 with the symptoms of **Sore throat/Congestion/Cough, SPO2:79, HRCT: 12/25** got cured following 3 Step Flu Diet in **4 days** under the N.I.C.E care of **Prateek Joshi**. After recovering completely, the patient was discharged on **03.06.2021**

Patient **Machindra Shinde** from **Jalkekhurud gaon, jalkekhurd** age **55** yrs, **Male,** was admitted in N.I.C.E Centre on **25.05.2021** with the symptoms of **Sore throat/ Breathlessness,:SPO2:77, HRCT:10/25** got cured following 3 Step Flu Diet in **5 days** under the N.I.C.E care of **Prateek Joshi**. After recovering completely, the patient was discharged on **03.06.2021**

Patient **Shivaji Hajare** from **Chinchala Tal- Mangrul, Dist- Washim, Chinchala** age **24 yrs** yrs, **Male,** was admitted in N.I.C.E Centre on **26.05.2021** with the symptoms of **Sore throat/ Cough** got cured following 3 Step Flu Diet in **4 days** under the N.I.C.E care of **Santosh Sarkale**. After recovering completely, the patient was discharged on **03.06.2021**

Patient **Ranjana Ramdas Bankar** from **kamargaon, kamargaon** age **60** yrs, **Female,** was admitted in N.I.C.E Centre on **25.05.2021** with the symptoms of **Chest Con-**

gestion/Cough HRCT:11/25 got cured following 3 Step Flu Diet in **4 days** under the N.I.C.E care of **Prateek Joshi**. After recovering completely, the patient was discharged on **03.06.2021**

Patient **Lata Chandrakant Rokde** from **karjule**, **karjule gaon** age **45** yrs, **Female,** was admitted in N.I.C.E Centre on **25.05.2021** with the symptoms of **Breathing Difficulty, SPO2: 88** got cured following 3 Step Flu Diet in **4 days** under the N.I.C.E care of **Prateek Joshi**. After recovering completely, the patient was discharged on **03.06.2021**

Patient **Poonam Yashwant Takle** from **radegan therpa**, **radegan therpa gaon** age **25** yrs, **Female,** was admitted in N.I.C.E Centre on **25.05.2021** with the symptoms of **Chest Congestion/Cough** got cured following 3 Step Flu Diet in **4 days** under the N.I.C.E care of **PrateeK Joshi**. After recovering completely, the patient was discharged on **03.06.2021**

Patient **Parvati Pawar** from **A/p- Mandavgan, Tal-Shirur Dist- Pune**, **Mandavgan** age **69 yrs** yrs, **Female,** was admitted in N.I.C.E Centre on **25.05.2021** with the symptoms of **Congestion, bodyache and weakness** got cured following 3 Step Flu Diet in **4 days** under the N.I.C.E care of **Santosh Sarkale**. After recovering completely, the patient was discharged on **03.06.2021**

Patient **Sindhu Uttam Ingle** from **panoli**, **panoli gaon** age **50** yrs, **Female,** was admitted in N.I.C.E Centre on **25.05.2021** with the symptoms of **Chest Congestion/ Cough** got cured following 3 Step Flu Diet in **4 days** under the N.I.C.E care of **Prateek Joshi**. After recovering completely, the patient was discharged on **03.06.2021**

Patient **Pradeep Uttam Ingle** from **panoli**, **panoli gaon** age **31** yrs, **Male,** was admitted in N.I.C.E Centre on **25.05.2021** with the symptoms of **Fever 101°F/Chest Congestion/Cough** got cured following 3 Step Flu Diet in **4 days** under the N.I.C.E care of **Prateek Joshi**. After recovering completely, the patient was discharged on **03.06.2021**

Patient **Manisha Anna Phulmadi** from **baburodi**, **baburodi gaon** age **17** yrs, **Female,** was admitted in N.I.C.E Centre on **25.05.2021** with the symptoms of **Fever 103°F/Chest/Congestion/Cough/Bodyache/Weakness** got cured following 3 Step Flu Diet in **5 to 7 days** under the N.I.C.E care of **Prateek Joshi**. After recovering completely, the patient was discharged on **03.06.2021**

Patient **Raju Dashrat Ajbe** from **kadhgaon**, **kadhgaon** age **48** yrs, **Male,** was admitted in N.I.C.E Centre on **25.05.2021** with the symptoms of **Chest Congestion/ Cough/Stomach ache** got cured following 3 Step Flu Diet in **4 days** under the N.I.C.E care of **Prateek Joshi**. After recovering completely, the patient was discharged on **03.06.2021**

Patient **Raosaheb Solji Kharmale** from **bhandgaon**, **bhandgaon** age **38** yrs, **Male,** was admitted in N.I.C.E Centre on **25.05.2021** with the symptoms of **:Fever 103°F/ Chest Congestion/Cough/Body Ache/Weakness, HRCT:10/25** got cured following 3 Step Flu Diet in **7 days** under the N.I.C.E care of **Prateek Joshi**. After recovering completely, the patient was discharged on **03.06.2021**

Patient **Kantabai Namdev Rode** from **klarjule gaon**, **karjule gaon** age **53** yrs, **Female,** was admitted in N.I.C.E Centre on **25.05.2021** with the symptoms of **Congestion/ Cough** got cured following 3 Step Flu Diet in **4 days** under the N.I.C.E care of Prateek Joshi. After recovering completely, the patient was discharged on **03.06.2021**

Patient **Kanu Bapu Phulmadi** from **baburodi**, **baburodi** age **30** yrs, **Male,** was admitted in N.I.C.E Centre on **25.05.2021** with the symptoms of **Congestion/Cough** got cured following 3 Step Flu Diet in **4 days** under the N.I.C.E care of **Prateek K Joshi**. After recovering completely, the patient was discharged on **03.06.2021**

Patient **Suman Adhav** from **At- Belwandi Tal- Shrigonda Dist- Ahmednagar**, **Belwandi** age **60 yrs** yrs, **Female,** was admitted in N.I.C.E Centre on **25.05.2021** with the symptoms of **Fever 102ºF, Headache, Bodyache, Chest congestion** got cured following 3 Step Flu Diet in **4 days** under the N.I.C.E care of **Santosh Sarkale**. After recovering completely, the patient was discharged on **03.06.2021**

Patient **Nilesh Adhav** from **At- Belwandi Tal Shrigonda Dist - Ahmednagar**, **Belwandi** age **37 yrs** yrs, **Male,** was admitted in N.I.C.E Centre on **25.05.2021** with the symptoms of **Fever 101ºF/ Headache/ Body ache/ Chest congestion** got cured following 3 Step Flu Diet in **4 days** under the N.I.C.E care of **Santosh Sarkale**. After recovering completely, the patient was discharged on **03.06.2021**

Patient **Santram Wagh** from **Karjule Harya Tal- Parner Dist - Ahmednagar**, **Karjule Harya** age **45yrs** yrs, **Male,** was admitted in N.I.C.E Centre on **31.05.2021** with the symptoms of **Breathing difficulty, weakness, head-**

ache, body ache, No smell got cured following 3 Step Flu Diet in **4 days** under the N.I.C.E care of **Santosh Sarkale**. After recovering completely, the patient was discharged on **03.06.2021**

Patient **Shyam T Patil** from **Adgaon**, **Parner** age **53** yrs, **Male,** was admitted in N.I.C.E Centre on **25.05.2021** with the symptoms of **Fever 104°F /Weakness/Body Ache/ Congestion/breathlessness, SPO2:86** got cured following 3 Step Flu Diet in **5 to 7 days** under the N.I.C.E care of **Amit Shimpi**. After recovering completely, the patient was discharged on **03.06.2021**

Patient **Yogesh Shyam Patil** from **Adgaon**, **Parner** age **30** yrs, **Male,** was admitted in N.I.C.E Centre on **25.05.2021** with the symptoms of **Fever 101°F /Weakness/Body Ache** got cured following 3 Step Flu Diet in **4 days** under the N.I.C.E care of **Amit Shimpi**. After recovering completely, the patient was discharged on **03.06.2021**

Patient **Janabai Pawar** from **Pokhari**, **Parner** age **66** yrs, **Female,** was admitted in N.I.C.E Centre on **28.05.2021** with the symptoms of **Fever102°F /Weakness/Body Ache** got cured following 3 Step Flu Diet in **4days** under the N.I.C.E care of **Amit Shimpi**. After recovering completely, the patient was discharged on **03.06.2021**

Patient **Kantabai khedekar** from **Parner**, **Parner** age **55** yrs, **Female,** was admitted in N.I.C.E Centre on **25.05.2021** with the symptoms of **Fever102°F /Weakness/Body Ache/Congestion/SPO2:83** got cured following 3 Step Flu Diet in **5 to 7 days** under the N.I.C.E care of **Amit Shimpi**. After recovering completely, the patient was discharged on **03.06.2021**

Patient **Suman Borghe** from **Vadegaon**, **Parner** age **55** yrs, **Female,** was admitted in N.I.C.E Centre on **26.05.2021** with the symptoms of **Fever103°F /Weakness/Body Ache** got cured following 3 Step Flu Diet in **5 to 7 days** under the N.I.C.E care of **Amit Shimpi**. After recovering completely, the patient was discharged on **03.06.2021**

Patient **Santosh Sakharam Pachpute** from **Taklidhokeshwar ,Tal partner dist Ahmednagar**, **Taklidhokeshwar** age **45** yrs, **Male,** was admitted in N.I.C.E Centre on **25.05.2021** with the symptoms of **Breathing difficulty/Weakness** got cured following 3 Step Flu Diet in **4 days** under the N.I.C.E care of **Vaishnavi Walunj**. After recovering completely, the patient was discharged on **03.06.2021**

Patient **Sangita Kane Phulmali** from **Bhalawani Ahmednagar**, **Bhalwani** age **28** yrs, **Female,** was admitted in N.I.C.E Centre on **25.05.2021** with the symptoms of **Dry Cough/ Chest Congestion/Body ache** got cured following 3 Step Flu Diet in **4 days** under the N.I.C.E care of **Vaishnavi Walunj**. After recovering completely, the patient was discharged on **03.06.2021**

Patient **Shashikala Bansi Matkar** from **Javkhade**, **Javkhade** age **62** yrs, **Female,** was admitted in N.I.C.E Centre on **25.05.2021** with the symptoms of **Dry Cough/ Chest congestion. She also has Blood Pressure issue** got cured following 3 Step Flu Diet in **4 days** under the N.I.C.E care of Vaishnavi **Walunj**. After recovering completely, the patient was discharged on **03.06.2021**

Patient **Sainath Govardhan Nimse** from **Kedgaon**, **Kedgaon** age **35** yrs, **Male,** was admitted in N.I.C.E Centre on **25.05.2021** with the symptoms of **Fever 100.2// Weakness/Body ache** got cured following 3 Step Flu Diet in **4 days** under the N.I.C.E care of Vaishnavi **Walunj**. After recovering completely, the patient was discharged on **03.06.2021**

Patient **Bhausaheb Heraji Dethe** from **Bolhegaon, Ahmednagar** age **53** yrs, **Male,** was admitted in N.I.C.E Centre on **25.05.2021** with the symptoms of **Dry Cough/ Chest Congestion/Body ache** got cured following 3 Step Flu Diet in **4 days** under the N.I.C.E care of **Vaishnavi Walunj**. After recovering completely, the patient was discharged on **03.06.2021**

Patient **Sushila Mahadeo Jadhav** from **Bhorwadi, Ahmednagar** age **72** yrs, **Female,** was admitted in N.I.C.E Centre on **25.05.2021** with the symptoms of **Fever 101.3°F/Body Ache/Weakness** got cured following 3 Step Flu Diet in **4 days** under the N.I.C.E care of **Vaishnavi Walunj**. After recovering completely, the patient was discharged on **03.06.2021**

Patient **Dattatray Bhikaji Borkar** from **Bhalavni, Ahmednagar** age **53** yrs, **Male,** was admitted in N.I.C.E Centre on **25.05.2021** with the symptoms of **Dry Cough/ Chest congestion, HRCT:7/25** got cured following 3 Step Flu Diet in **4 days** under the N.I.C.E care of **Vaishnavi Walunj**. After recovering completely, the patient was discharged on **05.06.2021**

Patient **Pratikche Dattatray Lahore** from **Kedgoan, Amednagar** age **19** yrs, **Female,** was admitted in N.I.C.E Centre on **26.05.2021** with the symptoms of **Weakness/ Sore throat** got cured following 3 Step Flu Diet in **4 days** under the N.I.C.E care of **Vaishnavi Walunj**. After recovering completely, the patient was discharged on **03.06.2021**

Patient **Sarjerao Kondiba Rithe** from **Bhalavni, Ahmednagar** age **55** yrs, **Male,** was admitted in N.I.C.E Centre on **25.05.2021** with the symptoms of **Fever 100.7/Dry Cough/Chest congestion** got cured following 3 Step Flu Diet in **4 days** under the N.I.C.E care of **Vaishnavi Walunj**. After recovering completely, the patient was discharged on **03.06.2021**

Patient **Baburao Khandu Kolpi** from **Bhalavni, Ahmednagar** age **25** yrs, **Male,** was admitted in N.I.C.E Centre on **25.05.2021** with the symptoms of **Dry Cough/ Chest Congestion/Body ache. He also has some psychiatric issues** got cured following 3 Step Flu Diet in **4 days** under the N.I.C.E care of **Vaishnavi Walunj**. After recovering completely, the patient was discharged on **03.06.2021**

Patient **Abasaheb Hari Bhau More** from **Mundhawa, Ahmednagar** age **35** yrs, **Male,** was admitted in N.I.C.E

Centre on **31.05.2021** with the symptoms of **Fever/ Breathlessness/Weakness** got cured following 3 Step Flu Diet in **4 days** under the N.I.C.E care of **Vaishnavi Walunj**. After recovering completely, the patient was discharged on **03.06.2021**

Patient **Laxmibai Govind Lanke** from **Nighoj**, **Ahmednagar** age **70** yrs, **Female,** was admitted in N.I.C.E Centre on **27.05.2021** with the symptoms of **Headache/Weakness, HRCT: 14/25** got cured following 3 Step Flu Diet in **4 days** under the N.I.C.E care of **Vaishnavi Walunj**. After recovering completely, the patient was discharged on **03.06.2021**

Patient **Jababai Bhau Thube** from **Pokhari**, **Ahmednagar** age **60** yrs, **Female,** was admitted in N.I.C.E Centre on **30.05.2021** with the symptoms of **Breathing difficulty, SPO2: 85** got cured following 3 Step Flu Diet in **4 days** under the N.I.C.E care of **Vaishnavi Walunj**. After recovering completely, the patient was discharged on **03.06.2021**

Patient **Vanita Vishal Chakale** from **Bhalvani**, **Ahmednagar** age **26** yrs, **Female,** was admitted in N.I.C.E Centre on **25.05.2021** with the symptoms of **Fever 99.3 F/ Weakness/Body ache** got cured following 3 Step Flu Diet in **4 days** under the N.I.C.E care of **Vaishnavi Walunj**.

After recovering completely, the patient was discharged on **03.06.2021**

Patient **Hausabai Sitaram rohokale** from **Bhalvani, Ahmednagar** age **70** yrs, **Female,** was admitted in N.I.C.E Centre on **31.05.2021** with the symptoms of **Fever and Weakness** got cured following 3 Step Flu Diet in **4 days** under the N.I.C.E care of Chitra **Jain**. After recovering completely, the patient was discharged on **04.06.2021**

Patient **Mane jalindar yedu** from **Mangrul, Ahmednagar** age **42** yrs, **Female,** was admitted in N.I.C.E Centre on **25.05.2021** with the symptoms of **Fever/Breathing difficulty, HRCT-15** got cured following 3 Step Flu Diet in **5 to 7 days** under the N.I.C.E care of **Vaishnavi Walunj**. After recovering completely, the patient was discharged on **03.06.2021**

Watch their video testimonial at
www.coronakaal.tv/delta72

Our Kissan N.I.C.E. Camp at Delhi (Ghazipur border) completed 100 days with No Mask, No PPE kit, No Sanitizer, No Oxygen cylinder, No Medication, No Fee and No Death

Our N.I.C.E. Experts (On 24X7 Duty)

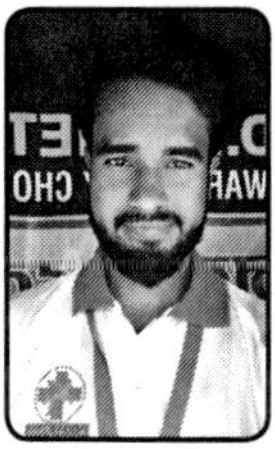

Raushan Kumar

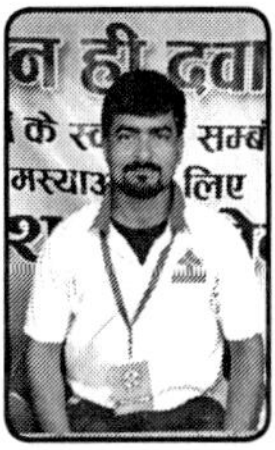

Sachin Kr. Singh

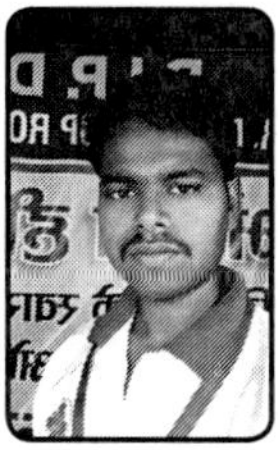

Dheeraj Gupta

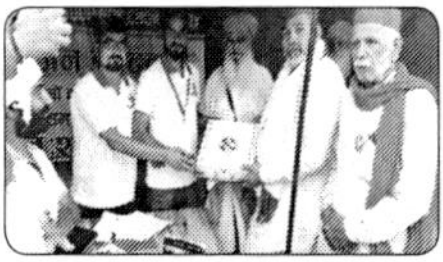

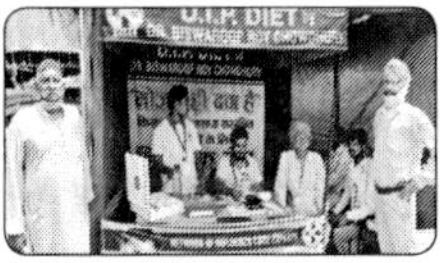

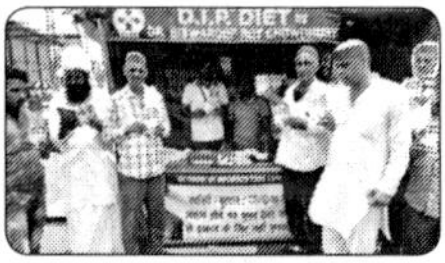

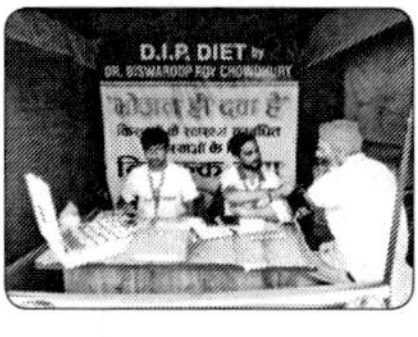

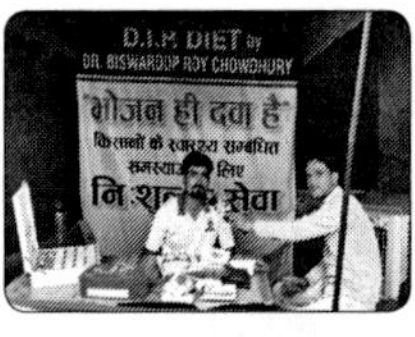

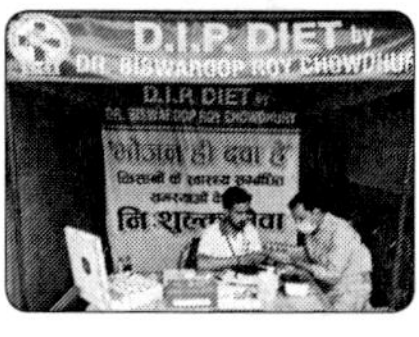

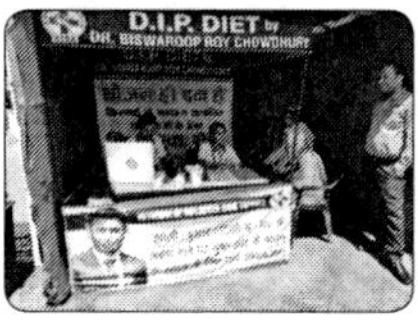

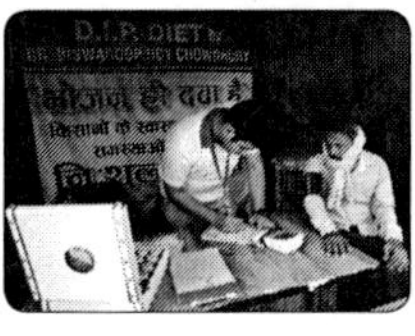

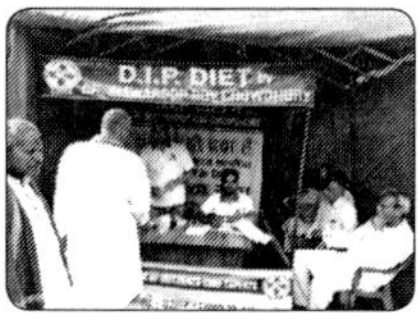

Our N.I.C.E. Team at Kissan N.I.C.E. Camp

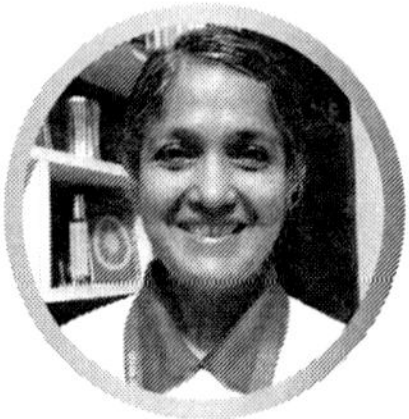
Seema Mannikoth

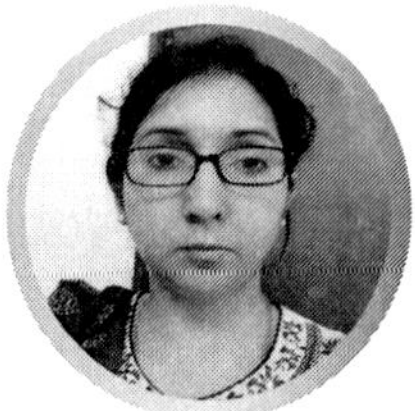
Dr. Shweta Chaudhary

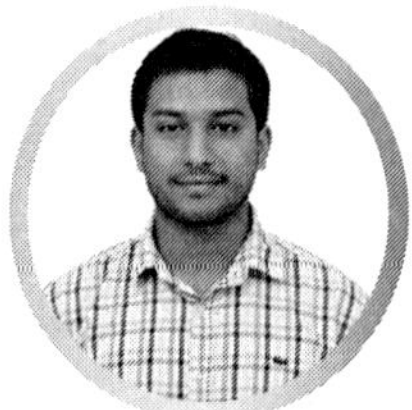
Harshit Maheshwari

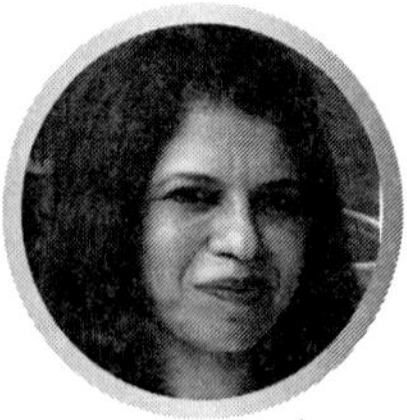
Hema Singh

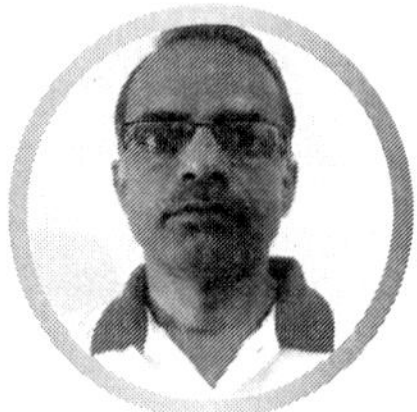
Jitendra Ramaiya

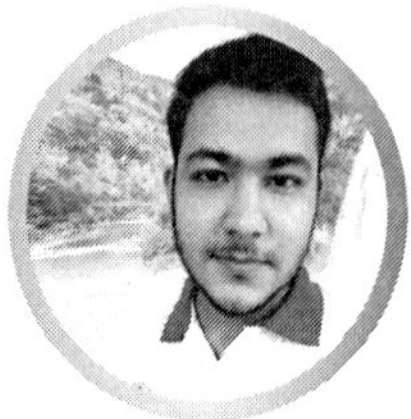
Kanishk Amarpuri

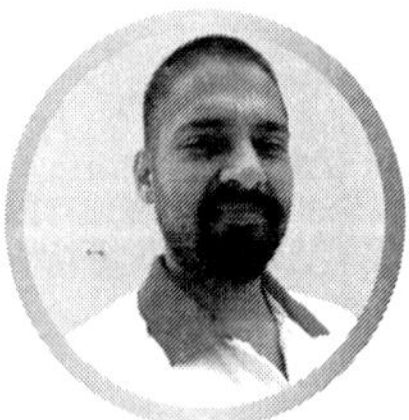
Manish Goel

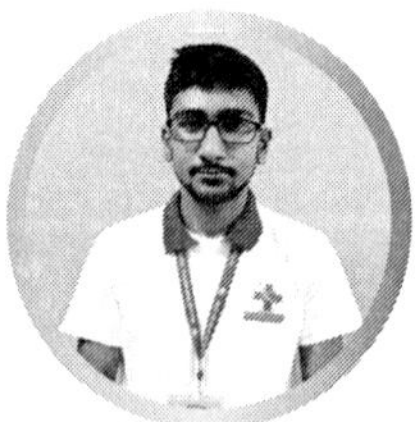
Manish Kumar Saini

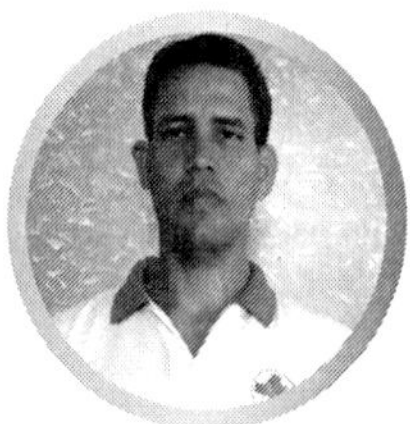
Mohit Vats

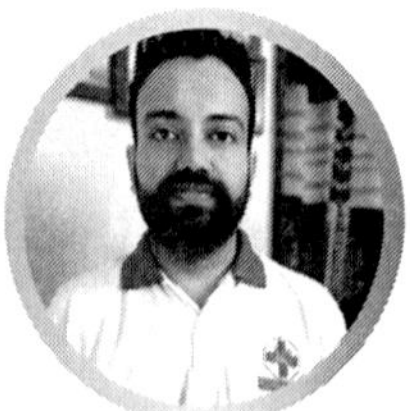
Pratik Anand

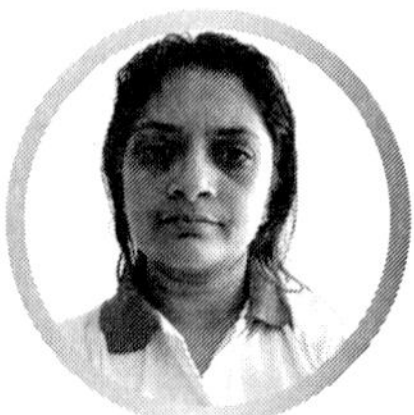
Richa Mishra

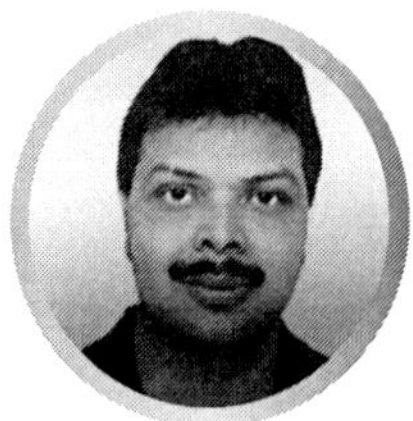
Sanjay Goopta

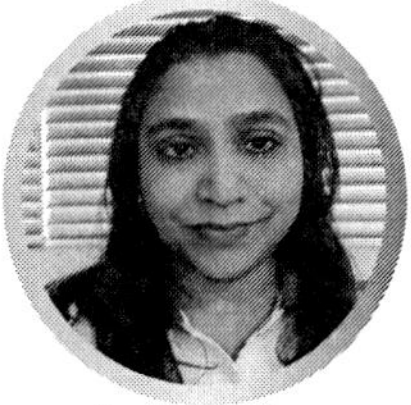

Amita Jain

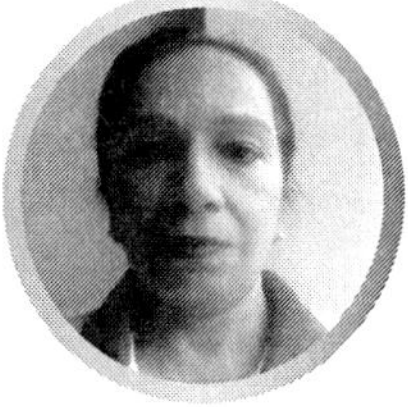

Simi Handa

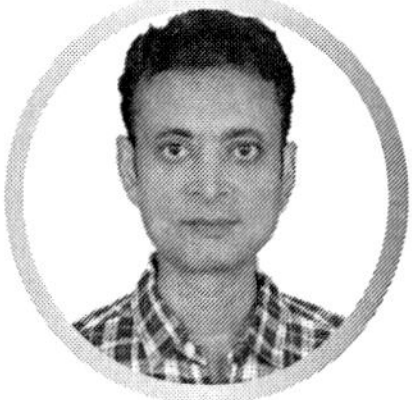

Sahil Mishra

Watch the video of Kissan N.I.C.E Camp at www.coronakaal.tv/kissancamp

Let every morning be the Hunza Morning

If you have decided to pick only one of my suggestions for the sake of your health, then take this suggestion:

Stop consuming tea specially, morning tea. The early morning tea makes the inner lining of your intestinal wall acidic, as after a long night of fasting your stomach is empty and craving for food. An acidic stomach on a regular basis is the single biggest cause of all kind of inflammatory and lifestyle diseases including arthritis, Diabetes etc.

How to stop craving of tea ⟶ Switch to Hunza Tea

Hunza Civilization: Hunza people are the Indians living at extreme northwest of India in Hindu Kush range. They are known to be one of the world's healthiest civilizations, often living up to the age of 110 years.

How to prepare Hunza Tea (serves four):

Ingredients:

- 12 Mint leaves(Pudina)
- 8 Basil Leaves(Tulsi)
- 4 Green cardamom (Elaichi)
- 2 gm Cinnamon (Dalchini)
- 20 gm Ginger (Adrak)
- 20 gm Jaggery (Gur)

Instructions:

- Take 4 cups of water in a tea pan
- Add all ingredients, simmer it for 10mins
- Add a dash of lemon juice and serve hot or cold